THERAPEUTIC EXERCISES SIMPLIFIED

FOUNDATIONS & TECHNIQUES WITHOUT THE GYM FOR FASTER RECOVERY, PAIN FREE MOVEMENT & LASTING MOBILITY TO REBALANCE YOUR BODY NATURALLY

SOLOMON CUNNINGHAM

CONTENTS

INTRODUCTION

Have you ever felt trapped by your own body, limited by pain or injury? You're not alone. Millions of adults struggle with physical challenges that hinder their ability to live life to the fullest. But what if there were a way to break free from these limitations and reclaim your strength? That's where therapeutic exercises come in.

This book is here to change the way you think about therapeutic exercises. It's not just for rehab after an injury. It's a powerful tool to help you build lifelong strength, resilience, and vitality. Whether recovering from a setback, looking to prevent future problems, or simply wanting to move better and feel stronger, this guide is for you.

We'll dive into the science behind therapeutic exercises and show you how they can benefit your body and mind. You'll learn practical strategies and techniques that you can start using right away. And we'll share real-life stories of people who have transformed their lives through movement.

But this book isn't just about the "how." It's also about the "why." We want to inspire you to see therapeutic exercise in a new light. It's not just something you have to do—it's something you get to do. It's a chance to take control of your health and well-being, to challenge yourself, and to grow stronger every day.

Throughout the pages of this book, we'll accompany you on this transformative journey. Our approach is to demystify the science of therapeutic exercise, translating complex theories into straightforward, accessible language. This book is free of overly technical terminology and intricate diagrams that might cloud your understanding. Instead, you'll find lucid, practical advice ready to be applied to your daily routine. Our goal is to make the principles of therapeutic exercise understandable and actionable for everyone, regardless of your starting point. Each chapter aims to equip you with knowledge and techniques that can be easily integrated into your life, fostering a deeper connection between you and your path to improved well-being. We'll start by building a strong foundation. You'll learn about the key principles of therapeutic exercise and how they apply to your unique body and needs. From there, we'll explore specific techniques and exercises that target different areas of the body. You'll discover how to modify movements to suit your current abilities and how to progress as you get stronger.

But this book isn't just a collection of exercises. It's a roadmap to a stronger, more resilient you. We'll show you how to integrate therapeutic exercise into your daily life so it becomes a natural part of your routine. You'll learn strategies for staying motivated, overcoming setbacks, and celebrating your progress.

By the end of this book, you'll have all the tools you need to make therapeutic exercise a lifelong habit. You'll feel stronger, more confident, and more in control of your health. And you'll be well on your way to reclaiming your strength and living the life you want.

So let's get started. Your journey to a stronger, more vibrant you begins now.

1

UNDERSTANDING THERAPEUTIC EXERCISE

———

Have you ever wondered why some people bounce back stronger after an injury while others struggle for months? The answer often lies in therapeutic exercises. This isn't just about doing a few stretches or lifting weights. It's about understanding how your body works and using that knowledge to heal and grow stronger. In this chapter, we'll explore what makes therapeutic exercises so effective. We will dive into the science behind it and see how it can change your life. You'll learn why therapeutic exercises are a key to not just recovery but long-term health and strength. Whether recovering from an injury or wanting to stay active and healthy, this chapter will give you the knowledge you need. We'll examine how therapeutic exercises work, why they matter, and how you can use them to feel your best daily. Let's start unlocking your body's power with therapeutic exercises.

1.1 THE SCIENCE BEHIND THERAPEUTIC EXERCISE

Therapeutic exercise works because of how it changes our bodies. When you exercise, your muscles adapt. They become stronger and more efficient. This happens because of muscle adaptation and hypertrophy. As you exercise, your muscles experience small tears. Your body repairs these tears, making the muscles stronger. This process is called hypertrophy. It is the reason why regular exercise leads to muscle growth and increased strength. But it's not just your muscles that change. Your brain also adapts. This is called neural adaptation. It helps you learn new movements and improve coordination. Through repeated practice, your brain creates new connections that make movements more straightforward and more natural over time. This is why once complex exercises become more straightforward to practice,

Blood flow and oxygenation also play a significant role. When you exercise, your heart pumps more blood to your muscles. This increase in blood flow brings more oxygen to the muscles, helping them work harder and recover faster. Oxygen is essential for muscle contraction, and increased circulation helps clear out waste products like lactic acid, which can cause muscle soreness. Hormonal responses are another critical factor. Exercise triggers the release of hormones like endorphins and growth hormones. Endorphins are often called the "feel-good" hormones because they improve mood and reduce pain perception. Growth hormone helps with tissue repair and muscle growth. These hormonal changes contribute to the positive effects of exercise on both physical and mental health.

Research supports the benefits of therapeutic exercises. Studies show that it improves outcomes in rehabilitation settings. For example, patients recovering from surgeries who engage in therapeutic exercises tend to regain function faster than those who do not. Longitudinal studies also show that regular exercise helps prevent chronic diseases like diabetes, heart disease, and obesity. Keeping your body active and strong reduces the risk of these conditions and improves your overall quality of life. Therapeutic and general exercises differ in their goals and methods. Therapeutic exercises focus on specific muscle groups and controlled, progressive loading. This means starting with light exercises and gradually increasing intensity. It ensures safe and effective recovery without risking further injury. Conversely, general exercise often involves broader goals like weight loss or general fitness without the same level of specificity.

Therapeutic exercises are a vital part of modern healthcare. It is often used alongside other treatments, such as medication or surgery. Physical therapists and doctors work together to create personalized exercise plans for patients. These plans address individual needs and ensure the best possible outcomes. Understanding how your body works and using therapeutic exercises can improve your health and help you recover faster from injuries. This chapter has shown you the science behind these exercises and how they make a difference. The following chapters will guide you in applying these principles to your life.

1.2 SHIFTING PERCEPTIONS: FROM RECOVERY TO VITALITY

Many see therapeutic exercises as a tool for getting back on track after an injury. But what if we considered it a way to stay ahead of the game? Imagine a world where exercise isn't just a reaction to a problem but a shield against future issues. This is not just about getting back to a baseline. It's about thriving. People often share stories of how regular exercise helped them stay healthy and avoid injuries. For example, a long-time runner who experienced knee pain avoided surgery by incorporating strength and flexibility exercises into his routine. This proactive approach kept him running for years.

Therapeutic exercises offer benefits that go well beyond physical healing. When you exercise, you often feel more precise and more focused. This happens because exercises improve blood flow to the brain, enhancing mental clarity. It also helps stabilize moods. Exercises can boost your mood and help you manage stress throughout the day. Regular movement builds resilience, making you less likely to get injured in the future. It also improves your overall health. Your heart strengthens, your metabolism works better, and your body becomes more efficient at using energy. These benefits contribute to a healthier, longer life.

As we grow older, maintaining vitality becomes crucial. Therapeutic exercises play a key role here. Balance and coordination exercises help prevent falls, a common concern for older adults. Simple activities like standing on one leg or walking heel-to-toe can make a big difference. Strength training supports bone health, helping to prevent conditions like osteoporosis. Lifting weights or resistance bands can strengthen bones and muscles, keeping them robust as you age. By incorporating these exercises, you support your body in staying active and healthy for years.

Seeing exercise as a lifestyle choice can transform how you live. It's not just something you do for a few weeks. It can become part of your daily routine. Many people start their day with a few minutes of mindful movement, such as gentle yoga or stretching. This kind of practice not only wakes up your body but also sets a positive tone for the day. You can also find ways to fit exercises into your daily activities. Try doing squats while brushing your teeth or stretching during TV commercials. These small changes add up, moving a natural part of your life.

Seeing exercises as a lifelong commitment rather than a temporary fix changes everything. It becomes a way to invest in your future health and happiness. By making therapeutic exercises a regular part of your routine, you empower yourself to live a fuller, more active life. You gain the strength to tackle daily challenges, the resilience to bounce back from setbacks, and the vitality to enjoy every moment. This approach to exercise is about embracing movement to enhance your life, not just fixing it when things go wrong. It's about living well for life.

1.3 KEY PRINCIPLES OF SAFE EXERCISE

Safety should always come first when you exercise. Proper form and alignment are key to avoiding injuries. Imagine bending to pick up a heavy box. If you use your back instead of your legs, you risk hurting yourself. The same is true for exercises. When you lift weights, keep your spine straight and your knees slightly bent. This helps distribute the weight evenly. Good alignment protects your joints and muscles from strain. It's like building a house. A solid foundation ensures the whole structure stays strong. Use mirrors or get feedback from someone experienced to check your form. Minor adjustments can make a big difference in your safety and effectiveness.

Warming up before exercise is as important as the exercise itself. Think of your body as a car on a cold morning. You want to let the engine warm up before you hit the road. A warm-up increases your heart rate and circulation. It prepares your muscles for activity— simple movements like marching in place or light jogging work well. After exercise, cooling down helps your body return to normal. Take a few minutes to stretch and breathe deeply. This reduces muscle soreness and helps prevent injuries. It also gives you a moment to reflect on your workout and appreciate the effort you've put in.

Listening to your body is another crucial aspect of safe exercise. Your body communicates in subtle ways. Learn to recognize the difference between pain and discomfort. Pain is sharp and persistent. It tells you something is wrong. Discomfort, on the other hand, is a sign of exertion. It's common when you push yourself a bit harder. If you feel pain, stop and reassess. Take a break or modify the exercise. Don't ignore fatigue, either. Your body needs rest to recover and grow stronger. If you're tired, adjust your routine or take a day off. Overtraining can lead to injuries and burnout.

Gradual progression is the cornerstone of any effective exercise plan. Pushing yourself to the limit is tempting, especially when you're eager to see results. But starting slow and increasing intensity carefully is crucial. Set realistic goals that you can achieve over time. Track your progress to stay motivated and avoid overexertion. Celebrate small victories along the way. They build confidence and momentum. Use a journal or app to note your achievements and challenges. This helps you stay on track and adjust your plan as needed. Remember, consistency beats intensity in the long run.

Finally, remember that exercise is not a one-size-fits-all solution. Your needs and goals are unique. Create a plan that suits your lifestyle and abilities. Assess your health conditions and limitations. This might mean consulting with healthcare professionals for personalized advice. They can help you design a program that targets your specific needs safely. For example, if you have knee pain, focus on low-impact exercises that strengthen your legs without putting stress on your joints. Use the right equipment and techniques to support your body. Adjust your plan as your needs change. Stay flexible and open to new approaches. Your body will thank you for it.

1.4 TAILORING EXERCISES TO INDIVIDUAL NEEDS

Understanding where you stand in your fitness journey begins with self-assessment. This step is crucial because it sets the foundation for your progress. To start, think about using self-assessment questionnaires. These tools help you evaluate your current fitness level. They ask simple questions about your activity routine, existing health conditions, and physical strengths and weaknesses. They give you a snapshot of your starting point. It's like checking your map before a road trip. You need to know where you are before you decide where to go. Another way to assess yourself is through basic physical tests. Try simple exercises that test your strength and flexibility. For example, see how many push-ups you can do or how far you can stretch your arms without discomfort. These tests provide a baseline to measure improvement over time. They also highlight areas where you may need extra focus or care.

When customizing exercises, consider any health conditions you have. Chronic conditions like arthritis or osteoporosis require special attention. For arthritis, low-impact exercises are ideal. Swimming or cycling can increase mobility without straining the joints. These activities keep you moving without the pounding impact of running or jumping. If you have osteoporosis, focus on weight-bearing exercises. Walking or light resistance training strengthens bones. It helps maintain bone density, which is crucial for preventing fractures. Modify exercises as needed to suit your comfort and capability. Always listen to your body. If something doesn't feel right, adjust the movement or try a different exercise that targets the same muscle group.

Different fitness goals require different approaches. If weight loss is your goal, incorporate high-intensity interval training (HIIT). These short bursts of vigorous activity burn calories efficiently. They keep your metabolism active even after the workout ends. Focus on activities that sustain your heart rate over time to build endurance. Activities like jogging, cycling, or brisk walking work well. They improve cardiovascular health and increase stamina. Adjust the duration and intensity to match your current fitness level. Gradually increase as your endurance builds. Tailoring your exercise routine to your goals ensures you work towards what matters most to you.

Adaptive equipment can make a big difference in your exercise routine. Resistance bands are versatile tools for varying intensity. Use them to add resistance to exercises like squats or bicep curls. The bands come in different strengths. Choose one that challenges you without causing strain or pain. You can also use stability balls to strengthen your core. These balls engage your muscles as you balance, providing an effective workout. They are great for exercises like crunches or planks. They add an extra challenge to your routine. They engage muscles you might not use with traditional exercises. Incorporating these tools can make your workouts more effective and enjoyable.

Tailoring exercises to fit your individual needs is a dynamic process. It requires awareness and adaptation. Your body is unique. Your exercise routine should reflect that uniqueness. Whether adapting to a health condition or working towards a specific goal, make your routine yours. Use the tools and techniques that fit your life and needs. Stay flexible and open to change. Adjust your routine as you learn more about what works for you. The journey to better health is personal. It evolves as you do. Embrace the process and make each step count.

Step 1: Starting Position

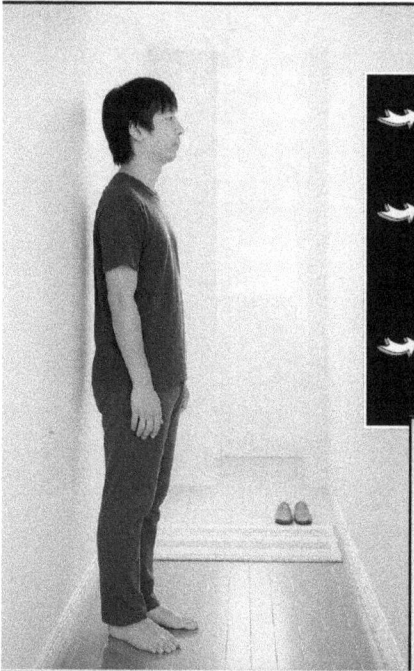

- Stand with your back against a flat wall.

- Place your feet shoulder-width apart, about 2 feet away from the wall.

- Keep your spine straight and shoulders relaxed.

- Slowly slide down the wall by bending your knees until they reach about a 90° angle.

- Ensure your thighs are parallel to the floor.

- Keep your back flat against the wall throughout the movement.

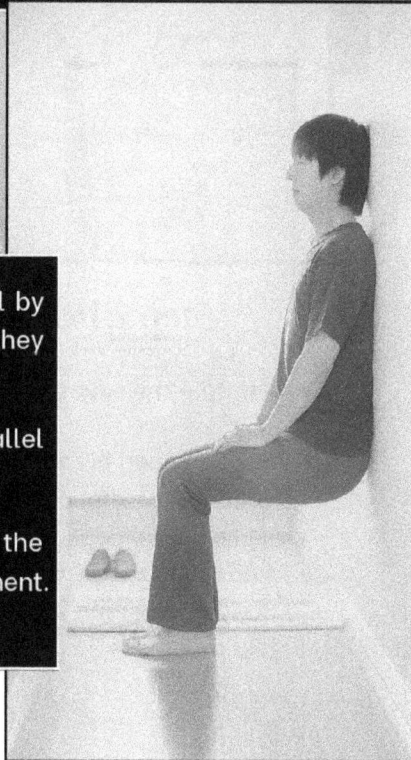

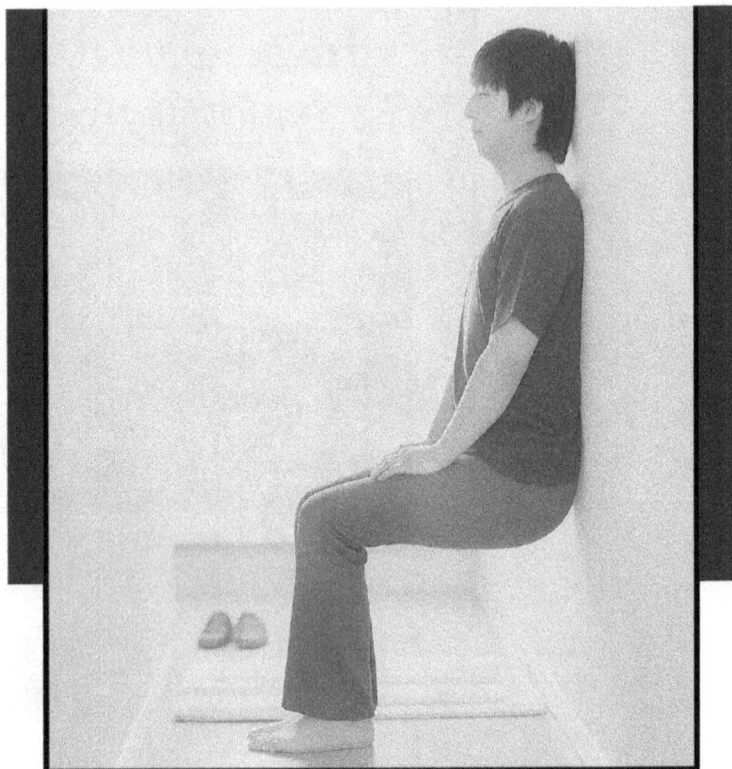

Step 2: Holding the Position

➥ Maintain the squat position, engaging your core.

➥ Practice deep breathing while holding the position. Focus on mindful alignment with each breath.

➥ Hold for 30 seconds and slowly rise back up to standing position.

1.5 THERAPEUTIC EXERCISES FOR MENTAL WELL-BEING

Exercise isn't just for the body; it also helps the mind. Many people find that regular movement reduces feelings of anxiety and depression. When you exercise, your brain releases chemicals that make you feel good. These chemicals, like endorphins and serotonin, help balance your mood. They also make you feel more relaxed. They can even help you sleep better. Studies show that people who exercise often feel less stressed and more in control of their lives. Exercise helps clear your mind, allowing you to focus better and think more clearly. This is why many people say they feel happier and more balanced when they stay active.

Some exercises are particularly good at boosting mental clarity. Mindful movement exercises combine movement with deep breathing, like yoga or tai chi. These exercises help you slow down and pay attention to your body. They teach you to focus on the present moment, which can reduce stress and improve mental sharpness. Breathing techniques also play a role. Deep, slow breaths calm the nervous system and lower stress levels. You can integrate these techniques into your routine by taking a few deep breaths before starting your workout. This helps set a calm, focused tone for your session. Over time, these practices can train your brain to stay calm and focused, even in stressful situations.

Real-life examples show how exercise can change lives. Many people have shared their stories of overcoming mental health challenges through exercise. Take the case of someone dealing with chronic anxiety. They started with short walks and gradually added other exercises, like swimming and yoga. Over time, they noticed they felt less anxious and more confident. Clinical studies support these personal stories. Research shows that exercise is an effective way to manage symptoms of depression and anxiety. In some cases, it works as well as medication. Exercise is a powerful tool that helps improve mental health and offers a sense of empowerment and control.

Exercises are also a great way to manage stress. Life is full of challenges, and stress is a natural response. But too much stress can be harmful. Exercise helps keep stress in check. When you move, your body releases tension and calms the mind. Short, daily routines can make a big difference. Even just ten minutes of stretching or dancing can reduce stress levels. Regular exercise builds resilience, making you better equipped to handle stress over the long term. It acts as a buffer, helping you bounce back from setbacks. This resilience spills over into other areas of life, making it easier to tackle challenges with a clear head and open heart.

Incorporating exercise into your life isn't just about getting fit. It's about finding balance and well-being. When you move a regular part of your routine, you support your body and mind. You create a foundation for better mental health and a happier life. So take a step towards a more active lifestyle, no matter how small. Every move counts, whether it's a walk in the park, a yoga class, or a few minutes of stretching at home. You'll feel better physically, and your mind will thank you, too. The benefits are waiting for you to unlock them. Movement is a path to a healthier, more balanced life, and it's never too late to start.

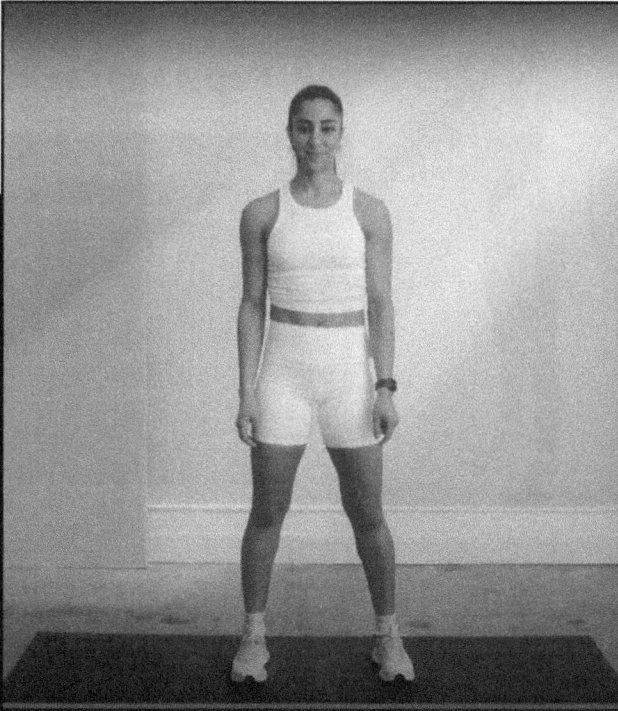

Step 1: Starting Position

🕊 Stand tall with your feet hip-width apart and arms by your sides.

🕊 Take a deep breath to center yourself and prepare for movement.

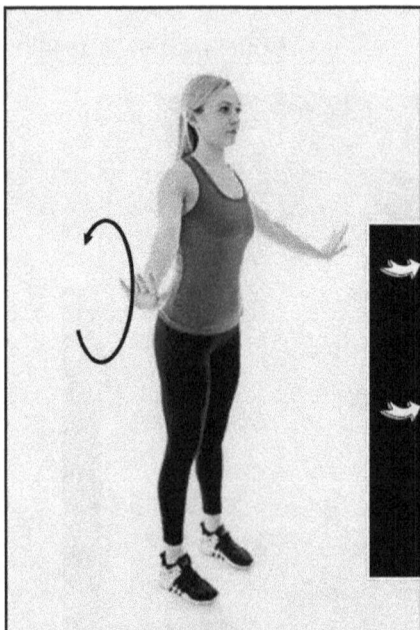

Step 2: Arm Circles

- Start by making small circles with your arms, gradually increasing the size.

- Perform this for 30 seconds, rotating forward, then switch to backward circles for another 30 seconds.

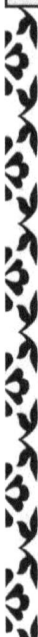

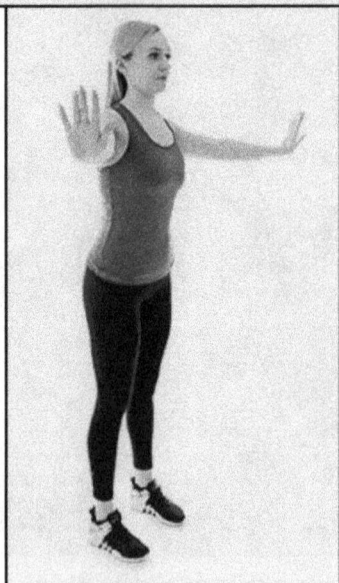

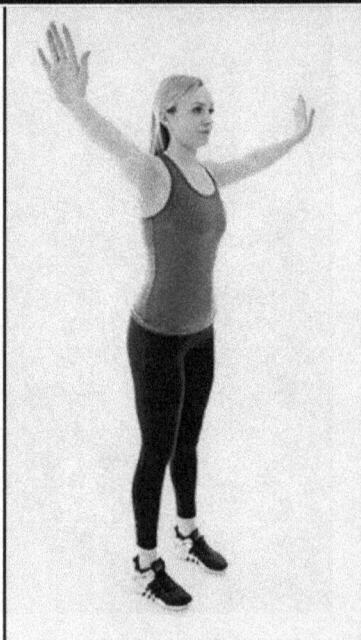

Step 3: Leg Swings

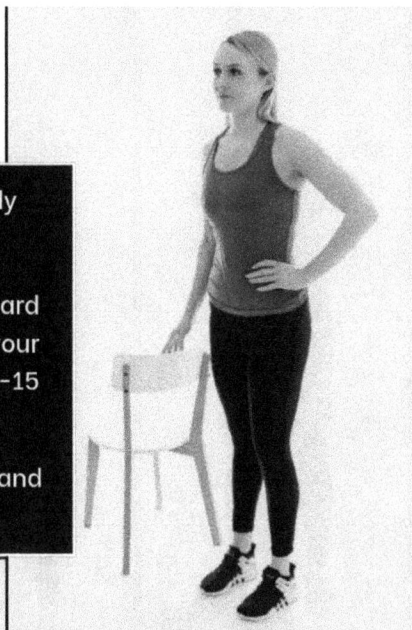

- Stand next to a wall or sturdy object for support.

- Swing your right leg forward and backward, keeping your posture upright. Perform 10-15 swings.

- Switch to the left leg and repeat the movement.

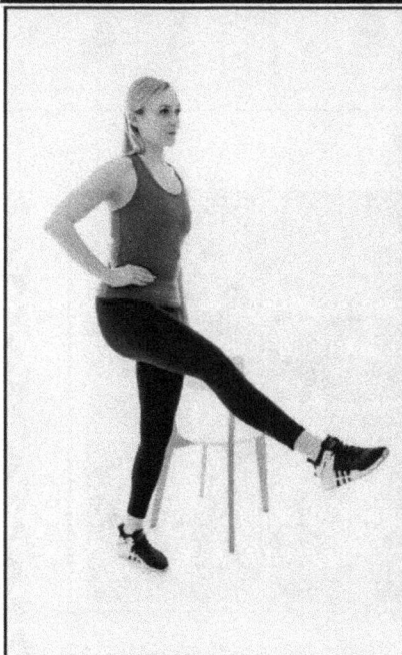

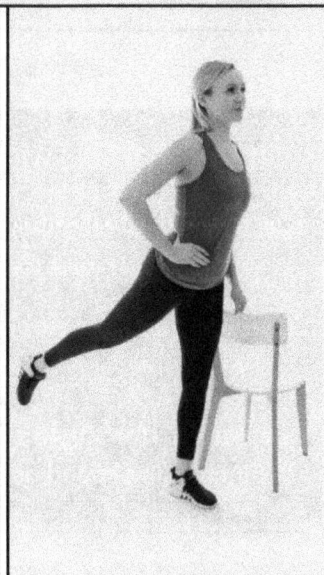

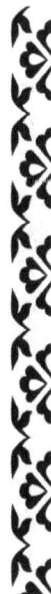

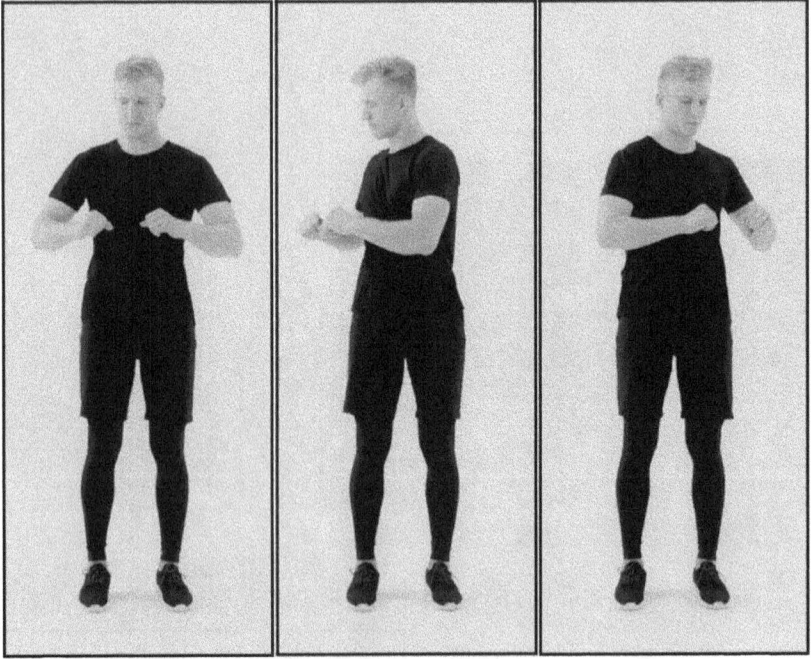

Step 4: Torso Twists

- Stand with feet shoulder-width apart and gently twist your torso to the right and left.

- Keep your hips stable while rotating through your spine.

- Perform for 30-45 seconds, gradually increasing speed as your body warms up.

2

BUILDING A STRONG FOUNDATION

———

I magine standing on a narrow log, trying to balance without falling. This simple act relies on one key part of your body: your core. Core stability is like the foundation of a building. It keeps everything upright and strong. When we talk about the core, we mean the muscles in your abdomen, back, and pelvis. These muscles work together to support your spine. They give you the balance and stability you need for almost everything you do. Whether picking up groceries, playing with your kids, or sitting at a desk, your core is working hard to keep you steady and safe.

A strong core does more than protect your back. It helps you move better and with more confidence. When your core is strong, you can lift objects more safely. This reduces the risk of injuries. Imagine bending over to lift a box. If your core is weak, you might strain your back. But with a strong core, your body stays aligned. This makes lifting more manageable and safer. Good core strength also supports better posture. When sitting for long periods, a strong core keeps your spine straight. This reduces stress on your lower back and neck, helping you feel more comfortable throughout the day.

Let's look at some exercises that improve core stability. Planks are a great place to start. To do a basic plank, lie face down, then lift your body so you're balancing on your forearms and toes. Keep your body in a straight line from head to heels. Hold this position for as long as you can. As you get stronger, try side planks. Balance on one forearm and the side of one foot, keeping your body straight. Another good exercise is the dead bug. Lie on your back with your arms and legs in the air. Slowly lower one arm and the opposite leg toward the floor, then bring them back up. Alternate sides. These movements engage your core muscles deeply and help build strength.

The bird-dog exercise is another effective way to target the core. Start on your hands and knees. Extend one arm forward and the opposite leg back, keeping your body stable. Hold for a few seconds, then switch sides. This exercise challenges your balance while working your core. It's simple but powerful. Doing these exercises regularly will help you build a strong and stable core. You'll notice improvements in how you move and carry yourself each day.

Some people think core exercises are the same as doing sit-ups or crunches. But there's a difference between core stability and abdominal exercises. Core stability involves the whole trunk, not just the abs. It includes muscles in the back, sides, and hips. These muscles work together to keep you balanced and stable. Abdominal exercises mainly focus on the front of the body. They don't provide the same comprehensive benefits as core stability exercises. Understanding this distinction helps you choose the correct exercises to meet your goals.

Building core stability is like laying a strong foundation for a house. It supports everything you do, making your movements more efficient and reducing the risk of injury. A strong core helps you live with more ease and confidence. When prioritizing core stability, you invest in a healthier, more active life. As you incorporate these exercises into your routine, you'll feel the difference in your daily activities. You'll stand taller, move more freely, and tackle challenges more easily. With a strong core, you're ready for whatever life throws.

Step 1: Starting Position

🕊 Begin on all fours, with your wrists directly under your shoulders and knees under your hips.

🕊 Keep your back straight and your neck neutral, looking down at the floor.

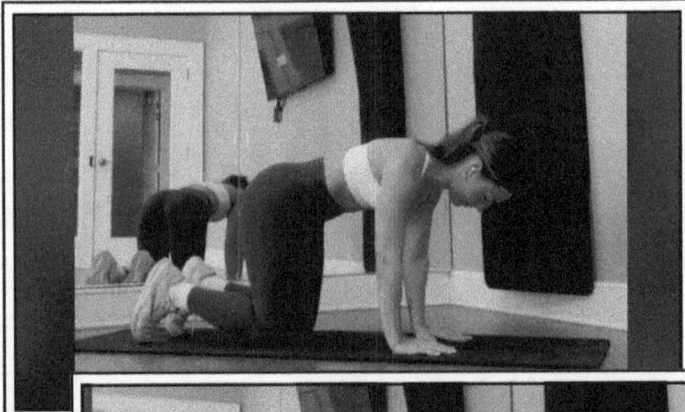

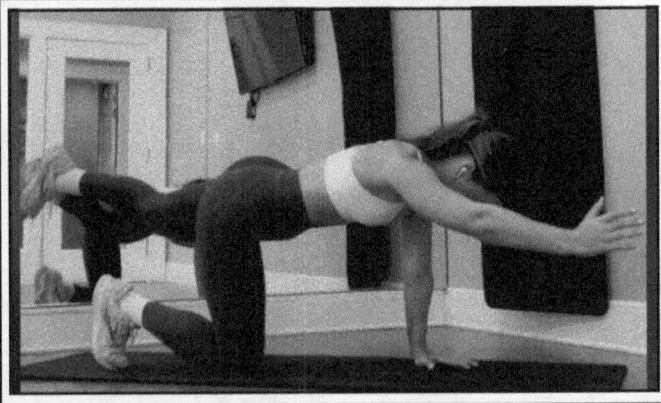

🕊 Extend your right arm straight forward and your left leg straight back, keeping both parallel to the ground.

Hold for 3 seconds, focusing on keeping your body stable and balanced.

Step 2: Tap and Return

Slowly bring your right hand and left knee toward each other underneath your body, tapping them lightly.

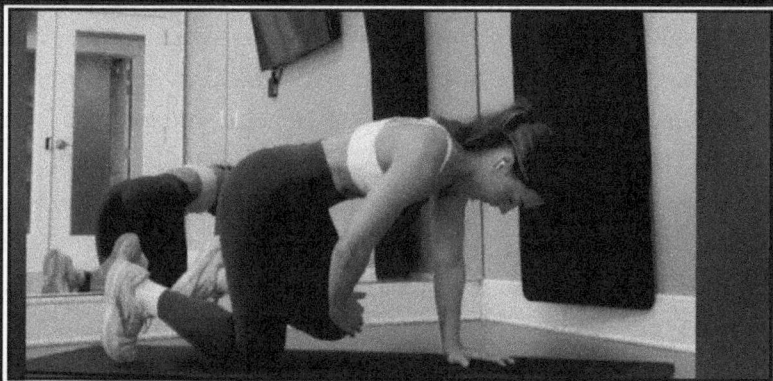

Extend your arm and leg back out to the starting position.

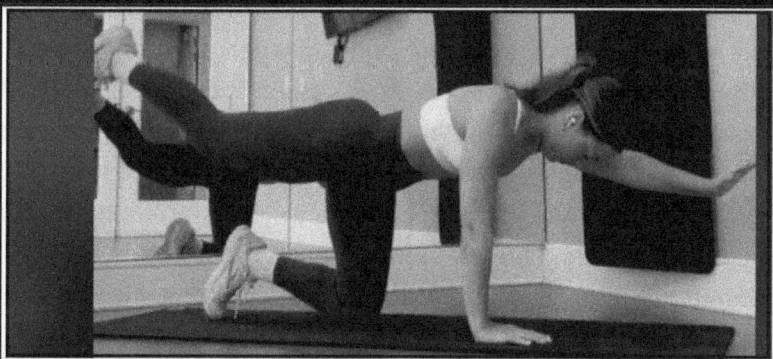

Repeat on the other side, alternating between each.

2.1 UNDERSTANDING RANGE OF MOTION (ROM)

Think about reaching for something on the top shelf or bending down to tie your shoes. These simple tasks depend on your range of motion (ROM). ROM is how far and how easily your joints can move in different directions. It's crucial for keeping your joints healthy and ensuring you move with ease. There are two types of ROM: active and passive. Active ROM is when you move a joint using your muscles, like lifting your arm. Passive ROM is when someone else moves your joint for you, like a therapist stretching your leg. Maintaining full ROM is essential because it helps you perform daily activities without pain or stiffness. When your ROM is limited, even basic tasks can become difficult. You might struggle to reach, bend, or twist, which affects your independence and quality of life. Restricted ROM can also lead to muscle imbalances and joint pain over time.

Improving your ROM can significantly affect how you move and feel. Dynamic stretching is a great way to enhance your ROM. Unlike static stretching, where you hold a position, dynamic stretching involves moving parts of your body through their full range of motion. This warms up your muscles and improves flexibility. Try arm circles, leg swings, or gentle lunges to start. Another effective technique is Proprioceptive Neuromuscular Facilitation (PNF) stretching. PNF involves stretching a muscle, contracting it, then stretching it again. This method increases flexibility by engaging your muscles more profoundly. You can practice PNF with a partner or on your own using a stretch-hold-relax pattern. These exercises improve joint function and help you move more freely.

When you work on your ROM, you also prevent injuries. Proper stretching keeps your muscles and joints flexible, reducing the risk of strains. It helps your joints stay lubricated, protecting the cartilage and keeping them healthy. This is especially important as you age or if you lead a sedentary lifestyle. Regular stretching and movement maintain joint health and prevent stiffness. Enhancing your ROM prepares your body for movement, reducing the chance of injury during exercise or daily activities. This preparation is like oiling a machine. It ensures everything runs smoothly and efficiently.

Assessing your ROM is a good way to understand your body's current capabilities. You can do simple tests at home to evaluate your ROM. For your shoulders, try reaching behind your head and touching the opposite shoulder blade. This checks your shoulder flexibility. For your hips, lie on your back and pull one knee towards your chest. This shows your hip flexibility. For your ankles, try the towel stretch. Sit straight and use a towel to pull your toes toward you. These tests give you a baseline to measure your progress. They help you identify improvement areas and track your development over time.

Understanding and improving your ROM is integral to maintaining your physical health. When you work on your flexibility and joint mobility, you support your body's ability to move efficiently and safely. This not only enhances your daily life but also helps you engage in more physical activities with confidence and ease. By incorporating ROM exercises into your routine, you take proactive steps toward preventing injuries and promoting overall well-being. Remember, your body's ability to move freely and without pain is a key component of a healthy, active lifestyle. Regular practice of these exercises will pay off in the long run, allowing you to enjoy the present and future activities you love.

2.2 PROPRIOCEPTION: ENHANCING BODY AWARENESS

Imagine walking into a dim room and instinctively knowing where the furniture is. This ability comes from proprioception. It's your body's way of sensing its position and movement in space. Proprioception plays a crucial role in exercise and daily life. It relies on sensory feedback mechanisms. These mechanisms help you adjust your movements and maintain coordination. Whether balancing on one foot or reaching for a cup, proprioception keeps you steady. It enables you to react quickly to changes in your environment. It's like having an internal GPS that guides your body through space. This sense is vital for maintaining balance. Good proprioception allows you to stay upright and stable, even on uneven surfaces.

To improve proprioception, engage in specific exercises. Balance exercises using stability balls are efficient. Your body must constantly adjust to stay balanced when you sit or lie on a stability ball. This engages your proprioceptive system, enhancing your body awareness. Single-leg stands are another simple yet powerful exercise. Stand on one leg while focusing on a point in front of you. Hold for a few seconds, then switch legs. This exercise challenges your balance and strengthens your proprioceptive ability. For a more advanced exercise, try using a wobble board. Stand on the board and shift your weight from side to side. This requires your body to make constant adjustments, further developing your proprioception.

Proprioception is key in injury recovery. When you improve your proprioception, you enhance neuromuscular control. This means your brain communicates more effectively with your muscles. Better communication leads to more coordinated movements and faster recovery. After an injury, your body needs to relearn how to move efficiently. Proprioception training accelerates this process. For example, exercises that challenge your balance help retrain your muscles and joints. These exercises reduce re-injury risk by improving your body's response to unexpected changes. Enhancing proprioception gives you greater control over your movements, which is crucial during rehabilitation.

In everyday life, enhanced proprioception offers many benefits. It allows you to navigate uneven terrain with confidence. Imagine hiking on a rocky path. With good proprioception, your body automatically adjusts to each step, keeping you stable. This reduces the likelihood of tripping or falling. Improved body awareness also boosts your confidence in physical abilities. You'll feel more secure when participating in sports or trying new activities. Whether you're playing tennis or dancing, proprioception helps you move gracefully and efficiently. It also makes daily tasks, like climbing stairs or carrying groceries, easier. With better proprioception, you become more in tune with your body, allowing you to react swiftly to any situation.

Incorporating proprioceptive exercises into your routine can transform how you move and feel. These exercises not only enhance your coordination but also boost your overall confidence. As you strengthen your proprioceptive sense, you'll notice improvements in balance, stability, and control. This newfound awareness empowers you to take on challenges with ease and assurance. By focusing on proprioception, you invest in a skill that benefits every aspect of your physical life. Whether recovering from an injury or seeking to improve your athletic performance, enhancing proprioception is a step towards a more capable and confident you.

2.3 FUNCTIONAL MOVEMENT PATTERNS

Consider the myriad of movements you engage in daily, from bending down to scoop up a child to exerting force to swing open a heavy door. At first glance, these activities might appear straightforward, yet intricate functional movement patterns underpin them. This concept revolves around exercises designed to mirror these commonplace actions, enhancing how you navigate daily life by making routine tasks more manageable. Functional movement training emphasizes exercises that utilize multiple joints and span various planes of motion, effectively engaging different muscle groups simultaneously. Rather than focusing on isolated muscle training, this approach advocates for a holistic regimen that trains the body to operate as a unified entity. Doing so fosters the development of strength, augments coordination, and optimizes overall movement efficiency. At the heart of functional movement are key patterns. Squat and hinge movements are essential. When you squat, you strengthen your legs and core. This helps in activities like lifting boxes or sitting in a chair. Hinge movements, like bending at the hips, protect your back. They teach you to lift with your legs, not your spine. This prevents strain when picking up heavy items. Push and pull actions are also crucial. A push movement, like a push-up, strengthens your chest and shoulders. It helps push a cart or open a door. Pull movements, such as pull-ups, work your back and arms. They help in activities like pulling yourself up or reaching for something above.

To reinforce these patterns, practice specific exercises. Goblet squats are a great start. Hold a weight close to your chest and squat down. Keep your back straight and knees aligned with your toes. This exercise improves leg strength and balance. Kettlebell swings are another effective movement. Swing the kettlebell between your legs, then up to shoulder height. This motion engages your hips, core, and shoulders. It builds power and endurance. For push patterns, try push-ups. Start on your hands and toes, lower your body, and push back up. This strengthens your chest, shoulders, and arms. Pull-ups are perfect for pull movements. Hang from a bar, pull your chin above the bar, then lower. This exercise targets your back and arms.

Understanding how well you perform these movements is essential. Functional Movement Screen (FMS) offers a way to assess your efficiency. FMS checks your ability to perform basic movements. It evaluates your balance, strength, and flexibility. This helps identify areas that need work. For example, you might score lower in a squat assessment. This could indicate tight hips or weak leg muscles. With this knowledge, you can focus on improving those areas. FMS provides a clear picture of how your body moves. It guides you in refining your technique and reducing the risk of injury.

Functional movement transcends the realm of conventional exercise, serving as a transformative approach to invigorating your daily life. Through the dedicated practice of these fundamental patterns, you elevate your proficiency in executing routine tasks and cultivate enhanced strength and seamless coordination. This newfound prowess significantly simplifies lifting, pushing, and pulling activities, thereby streamlining your day-to-day experiences and infusing them with greater ease and enjoyment. By weaving functional movement exercises into your daily regimen, you'll observe a noticeable shift in your movement efficiency and overall physical sensation—a testament to your body's gratitude for embracing a practice that aligns with its natural mechanics and needs.

2.4 BIOMECHANICS FOR INJURY PREVENTION

Understanding biomechanics is like knowing the blueprint of your body. It tells you how your muscles, bones, and joints work together to make you move. When you understand this, you can prevent injuries and move more efficiently. The key is in alignment and force distribution. Imagine your body as a machine. If one part is out of place, the whole system struggles. Keeping your body aligned is crucial. It ensures that forces are evenly distributed across your muscles and joints. This reduces the risk of wear and tear. When you lift something heavy, proper alignment protects your spine and muscles. It prevents strains and injuries that occur when you lift with poor form.

Levers and muscle action also play a significant role in biomechanics. Your body uses levers to move. Think of your arm as a lever. Your elbow is the pivot point. Your muscles apply force to move your arm. Understanding this helps you use your muscles more efficiently and avoid overloading any one part of your body. For example, when lifting weights, engaging the right muscles and using proper technique protects your joints. This way, you lift safely and effectively, reducing injury risks.

Common biomechanical errors often lead to injuries. Poor lifting techniques are a frequent culprit. Many people lift with their backs instead of their legs. This strains the lower back and can cause serious injuries over time. Always remember to bend your knees and keep your back straight when lifting. Another common mistake is incorrect running form. Many runners land heavily on their heels, causing shock to travel up the legs. This can lead to stress fractures and joint pain. Running with a mid-foot strike and keeping your body upright can help prevent these issues. Minor adjustments in form can make a big difference in how you feel and perform.

To better understand your movement patterns, consider biomechanical assessments. Gait analysis is a valuable tool. It examines how you walk or run. This analysis helps identify any imbalances or inefficiencies in your movement. A physical therapist or trained professional can perform this assessment. They provide insights into how to improve your form. Video analysis is another method. Record yourself performing exercises or daily activities. Watch the playback to spot any issues with alignment or technique. This visual feedback is invaluable for making necessary corrections.

Improving biomechanics requires targeted exercises and strategies. Focus on strengthening exercises that support proper posture. Exercises like rows and back extensions strengthen the muscles that support your spine. This helps maintain good alignment during activities. Flexibility routines also play a part. Stretching imbalanced muscles ensures they work in harmony. Regularly stretch your hamstrings, hip flexors, and shoulders. This keeps your muscles flexible and reduces the risk of injury. Incorporating these exercises into your routine improves your overall biomechanics. It helps you move more efficiently and with less risk of injury. Understanding biomechanics empowers you to take control of your movement. It allows you to exercise safely and effectively, supporting a healthier, more active lifestyle.

By focusing on these elements of biomechanics, you create a foundation for safe and efficient movement. Each part of your body works together to function as a whole. When you understand and apply these principles, you prevent injuries and move with confidence. These insights help not only with exercise but also with daily life tasks. Moving well means living well. As you build on this foundation, you'll be ready to explore more advanced techniques and strategies in the next chapter.

Step 1: Starting Position

🪶 Stand with feet hip-width apart and arms extended out to your sides for balance.

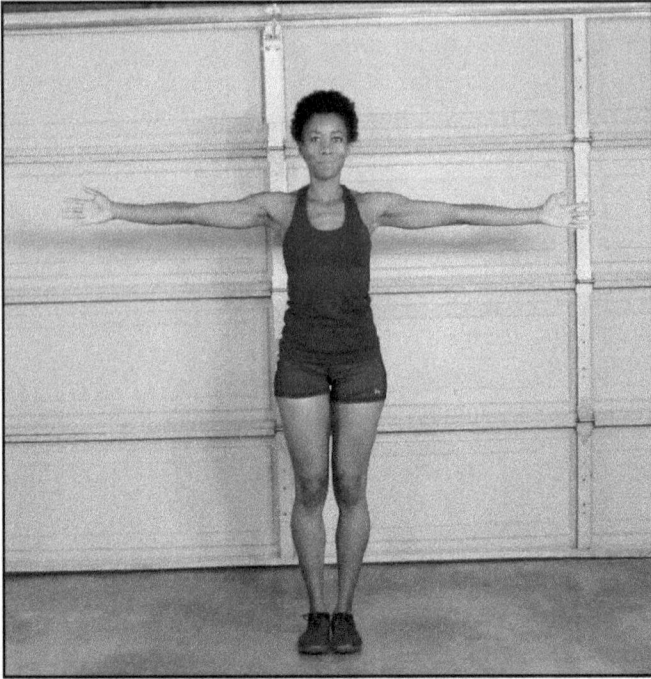

Step 2: Single-Leg Balance

🪶 Lift your right leg off the ground, bending it slightly at the knee, and balance on your left leg.

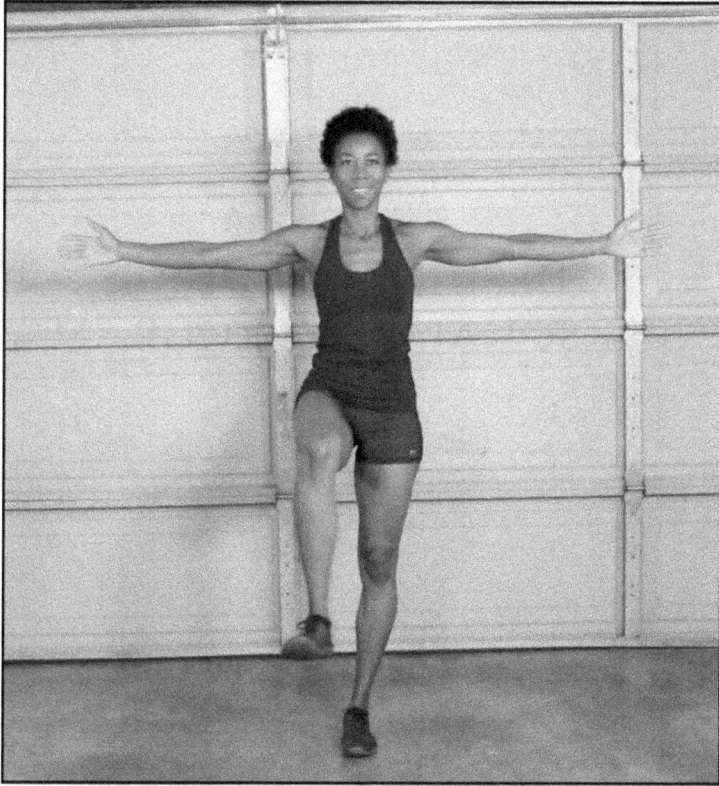

➤ Hold for 20-30 seconds, keeping your hips stable and engaging your core.

➤ Focus on controlled movement and maintaining proper posture throughout the exercise.

➤ Switch to the other leg and repeat.

3
DESIGNING YOUR PERSONALIZED PROGRAM

———

Have you ever tried to assemble a puzzle without seeing the picture on the box? It can be confusing and frustrating. Designing a personalized exercise program can feel the same way. You need to know where each piece fits to see the whole picture. This chapter is about helping you find those pieces. It starts with understanding where you stand right now. You must assess your fitness level, health conditions, and what you want to achieve. This isn't just about knowing where you're strong. It's also about spotting areas where you can improve.

Begin with a comprehensive self-assessment. This means looking at what you can do physically and where to improve. Try simple physical tests to check your endurance and flexibility. How long can you hold a plank? How far can you stretch your arms? These tests give you a clear idea of your current level. They help you see where you excel and where you need more work. Health questionnaires also play a key role. They ask about your medical history and any conditions you have. This helps you figure out what exercises are safe and effective for you.

Recognize your strengths and limitations. This is crucial for designing a program that works. Everyone has areas where they excel and others where they struggle. Look for muscle imbalances that might cause strain or injury. Source 2 explains that imbalances often lead to pain and stiffness. You can focus on exercises that help balance your muscles by identifying them. Also, consider your cardiovascular capacity. Can you walk briskly for 20 minutes without feeling winded? Knowing this helps tailor your exercise intensity.

After gathering your baseline data, it's time to craft realistic and personalized goals. Goals serve as beacons of motivation and direction on your fitness journey. Begin by setting short-term objectives that are attainable within a brief period. For instance, you might aim to enhance your flexibility within a month. Once achieved, this immediate goal provides a clear target and a sense of accomplishment. Following this, establish long-term goals for continued progress. These ambitions should stretch your capabilities further, such as completing a 5k run in six months. The key to practical goal setting lies in its specificity and feasibility. To structure your goals effectively, employ the SMART criteria: Specific, Measurable, Achievable, Relevant, and Timely. This method ensures that each goal has a clear definition and outcome. A 'Specific' goal narrows down precisely what you aim to achieve, offering more clarity than a vague aim.

Making your goal 'Measurable' means setting tangible benchmarks to gauge progress, such as timing a run or counting repetitions. 'Achievable' ensures that, while challenging, the goal is within the bounds of possibility, considering your current abilities and constraints. 'Relevant' goals align with your broader aspirations and motivations, ensuring that each milestone is a step towards a larger purpose.

Finally, 'Timely' goals have defined deadlines, creating urgency and helping prioritize efforts. This strategic methodology does more than clarify your objectives; it significantly boosts motivation by charting a course filled with attainable milestones. As you journey through your fitness regimen, it's imperative to reassess and recalibrate these goals periodically. This dynamic process allows your objectives to evolve with your increasing capabilities, fostering an ongoing cycle of motivation and success. By continuously setting, achieving, and then setting new, more challenging goals, you ensure that your fitness journey is marked by constant growth and improvement. This approach keeps you engaged and motivated and celebrates your progress, making the path toward wellness both rewarding and enjoyable. Use assessment tools and resources to track your progress. Like those mentioned in Source 1, fitness tracking apps provide valuable insights. They help you monitor your workouts and see improvements over time. Apps like Nike Training Club offer a variety of classes and are great for tracking progress. Wearable technology, like fitness watches, can also be helpful. They track your heart rate and activity levels. This data helps you adjust your program as needed. Professional fitness assessment kits offer more detailed insights. They often include tools to measure body composition and flexibility. This information helps you fine-tune your program for even better results.

Assessing your starting point is like drawing a map for your fitness journey. It helps you see where you are and where you want to go. By understanding your strengths and limitations, you create a personalized program that fits your needs. Use the tools available to track your progress and adjust as you go. This approach not only brings you closer to your goals but also makes the process enjoyable and rewarding.

3.1 DEVELOPING A PERSONALIZED EXERCISE PLAN

Creating an exercise plan is like designing a blueprint for your health. It requires careful thought and planning. Start by outlining a structured framework that fits your goals. This means considering how often you can realistically work out each week. Aim to balance different exercise types in your schedule. You can do strength training on Mondays and Thursdays. Then, reserve Tuesdays for flexibility exercises and Saturdays for cardiovascular activities. Always include rest and recovery days. These are just as important as workout days. They allow your muscles to heal and grow stronger. Overworking yourself can lead to fatigue and injury, so listen to your body and adjust when needed.

Variety in your exercise routine keeps things interesting and targets different aspects of fitness. Strength training helps build muscles and supports your joints. It can be as simple as lifting weights or using resistance bands. Flexibility exercises improve your range of motion and reduce the risk of injury. Activities like yoga or stretching routines are great for this. Cardiovascular activities, like walking or cycling, improve heart health and increase stamina. Mixing these types of exercises ensures you work on all areas of fitness. This balanced approach keeps you engaged and helps you develop a well-rounded fitness level.

Everyone's body is different, and health issues can affect how you exercise. For instance, if you have joint pain, look for exercises that are gentle on your joints. Swimming or using an elliptical machine are excellent options. They provide a good workout without putting too much stress on your knees or hips. If you have cardiovascular limitations, start with short sessions to build endurance. Gradually increase the time and intensity as your fitness improves. Tailoring your plan to accommodate any health conditions ensures you exercise safely and effectively. It also makes the experience more enjoyable and less daunting.

Your lifestyle plays a significant role in designing your exercise plan. Time management is crucial, especially if you have a busy schedule. Look for small pockets of time to fit in your workouts. You could do a quick session during your lunch break or right after work. Setting up a home exercise area can also save you time. You don't need a lot of space or equipment. Just make sure you have enough room to move freely. Keep your exercise gear handy to start your workout without any hassle. This convenience makes it easier to stick to your routine.

Step 1: Starting Position

↪ Stand tall with feet shoulder-width apart and arms by your sides.

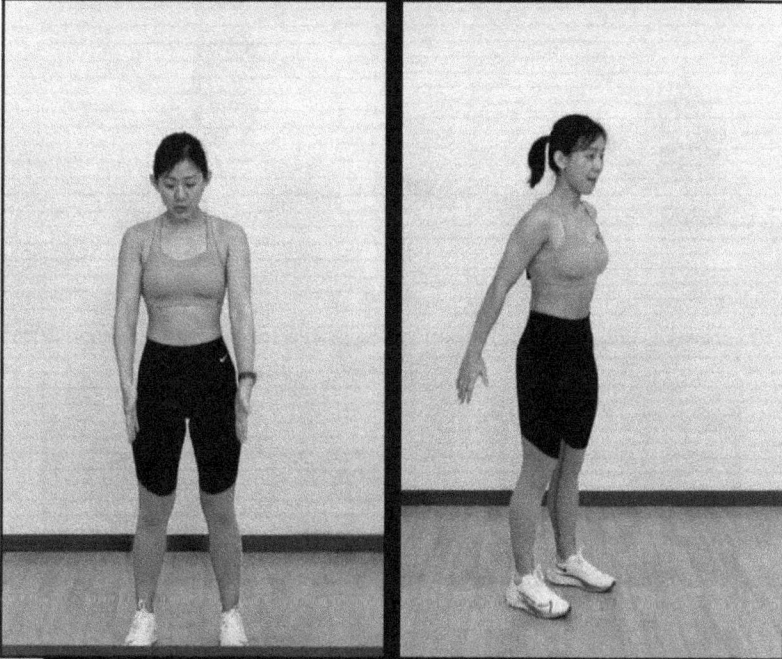

Step 2: First Exercise – Squats

↪ Slowly bend your knees and lower your body until your thighs are parallel to the floor.

↪ Push through your heels to return to standing.

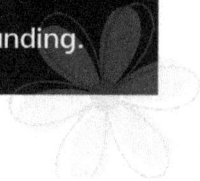

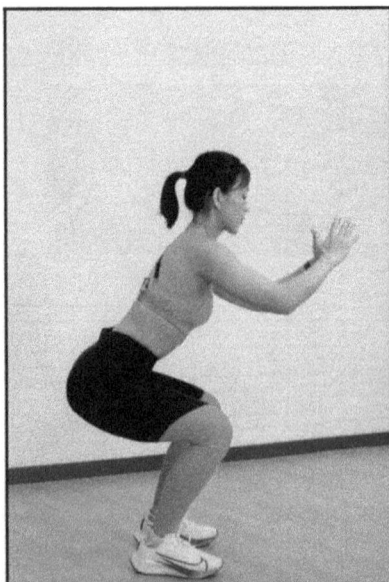

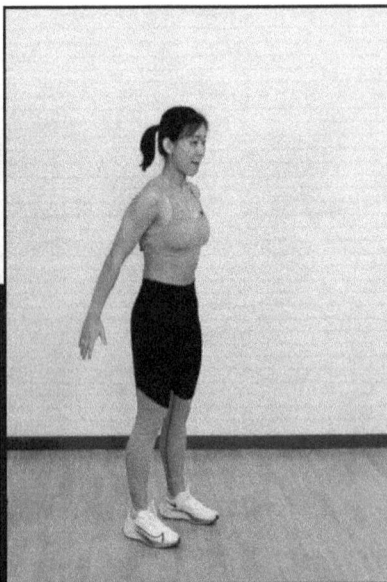

> Perform 10-12 reps.

Step 3: Second Exercise – Push-Ups

> Start in a plank position, hands shoulder-width apart.

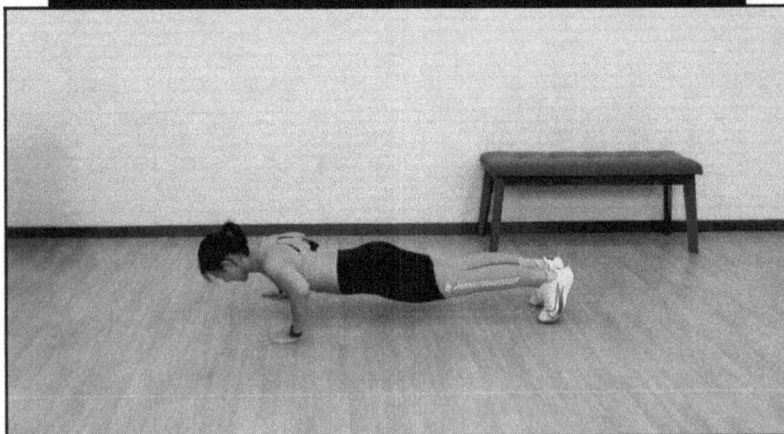

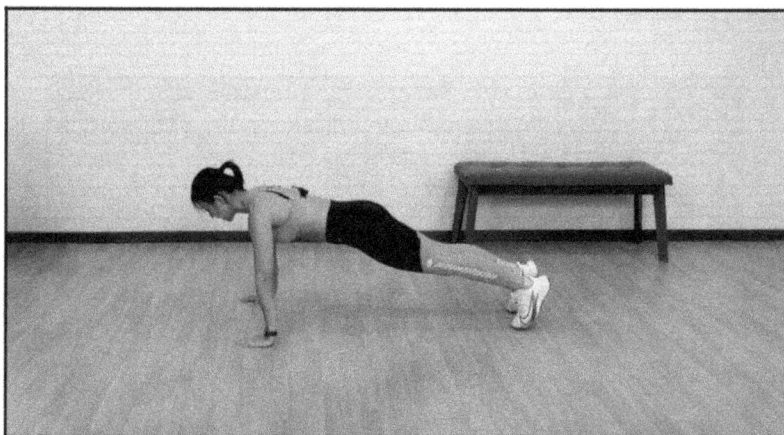

Perform 8-10 reps (modify by doing it on your knees if necessary).

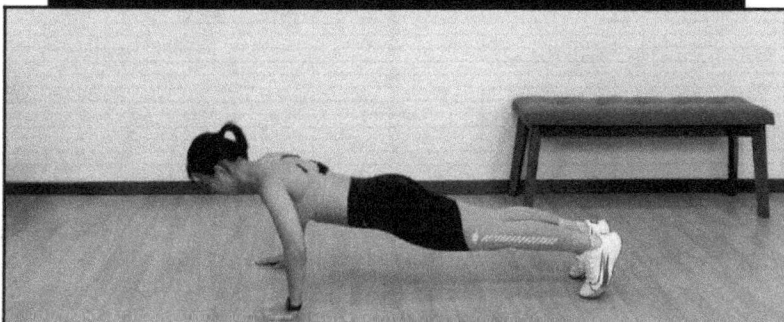

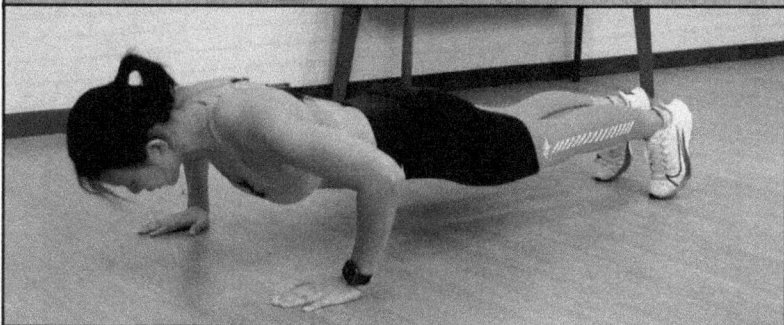

Step 4: Third Exercise – Lunges

➤ Step forward with one leg, lowering your body until both knees are at 90° angles.

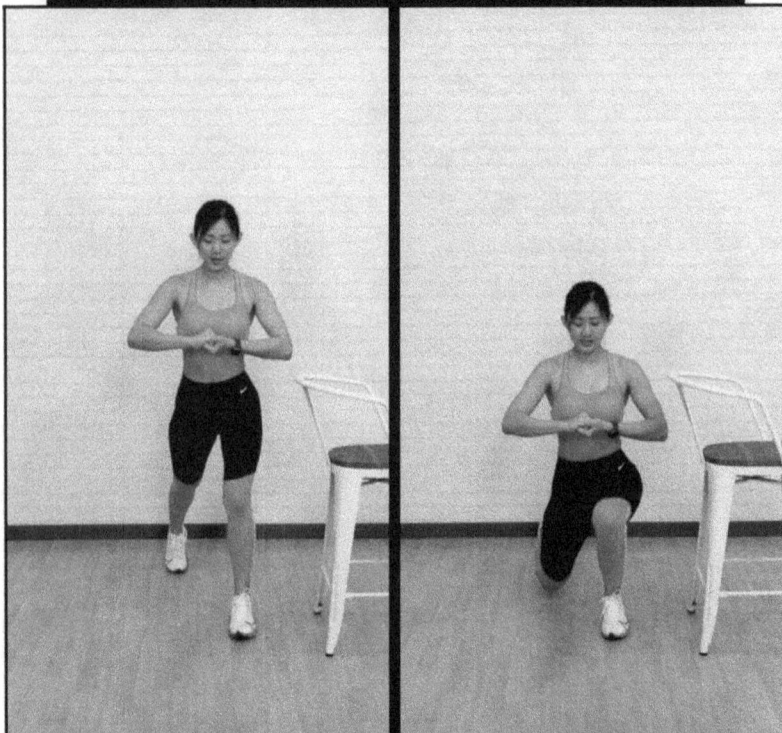

➤ Push through the front heel to return to standing and repeat on the other leg.

➤ Perform 8-10 reps per leg.

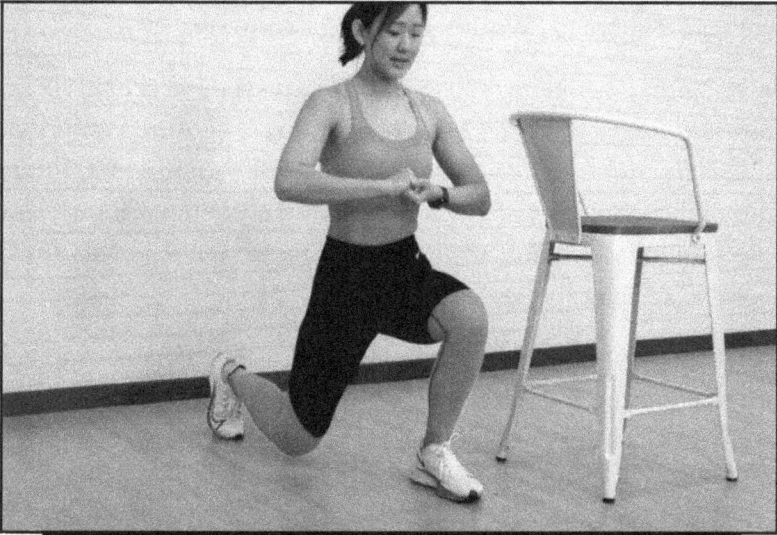

Step 5: Fourth Exercise – Plank

🐦 Hold a forearm plank position with a straight line from head to heels.

🐦 Hold for 30-45 seconds.

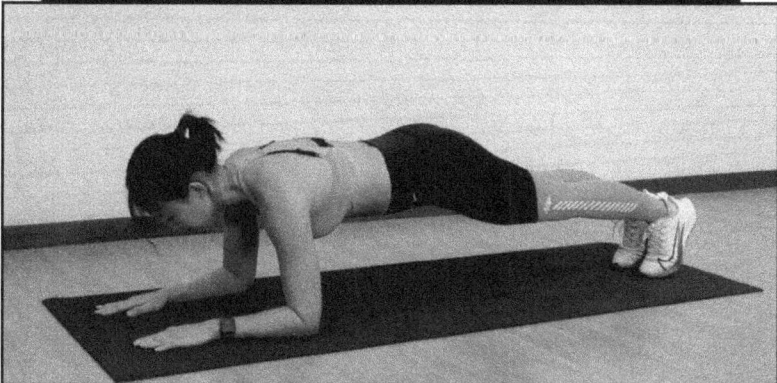

Interactive Element: Weekly Planning Template

Use a planning template to help you organize your week. This simple tool lets you map out your workouts and rest days. Write down your exercise type for each day and the time you'll dedicate to it. Include notes on how you feel after each session. This helps you track your progress and make adjustments when needed. Having a visual plan keeps you accountable and motivated.

Remember, your exercise plan should fit into your life, not vice versa. Consider your daily commitments and energy levels. Be flexible and willing to adjust your schedule as needed. Some days, you might feel too tired for a high-intensity workout. That's okay. Swap it for a light walk or stretching session. The key is consistency and making exercise a natural part of your routine. By crafting a plan that aligns with your goals and lifestyle, you set yourself up for success.

3.2 TRACKING PROGRESS AND ADJUSTING GOALS

Keeping track of your progress is like keeping a diary of your fitness life. It helps you see where you've been and where you are heading. One of the most effective ways to do this is by maintaining a detailed exercise journal. Each day you work out, jot down what you did, how long you did it, and how you felt afterward. This might seem simple, but it provides a wealth of information. Over time, you'll notice patterns. You may feel more energized after morning workouts, or you may see improvements in your mood after yoga sessions. This written record becomes a map of your journey, showing how far you've come and helping you plan where to go next.

Digital tools also play a huge role in tracking progress. Many apps make this process easy and even fun. Apps like Nike Training Club or Strava let you log workouts, track distance, and even set reminders for your next session. They also offer visual charts and graphs, making it easy to see your progress at a glance. You can track your strength gains and endurance levels and even monitor your heart rate. These insights are not just numbers. They tell a story of your growth and help you stay motivated. They prove that your hard work is paying off, even when you might not feel it.

As you track your progress, it's essential to recognize the signs of improvement. Increased stamina is one of the first things you might notice. Activities that once left you breathless become easier. You could walk up a flight of stairs without stopping or lift heavier weights than before. These physical changes are exciting and motivating. But don't forget about the mental benefits. Many people find that regular exercise enhances their mood and mental clarity. You might feel less stressed and more focused. You might even notice a boost in confidence. Celebrate these achievements. They are essential landmarks on your fitness path.

Adjusting your goals as you progress is crucial. Once you hit a milestone, set a new challenge. This keeps your workout routine fresh and engaging. For instance, if you've been walking 10,000 steps daily, challenge yourself to add 1,000 steps. Or, if you've mastered a basic yoga pose, try a more advanced version. Regular goal reassessment helps you stay focused and motivated. It also prevents you from getting stuck in a routine that no longer challenges you. Remember, fitness is not a destination. It's about continuous improvement and growth.

Feedback is another valuable tool for improvement. Take time for self-reflection and check-ins. Ask yourself what is working and what isn't. Are there exercises you dread? It may be time to swap them for something you enjoy more. Consult with fitness professionals if possible. They can offer an outsider's perspective and suggest tweaks to your program. This might include adjusting your form or trying new exercises. Professional feedback can provide insights that you might overlook on your own. It's like having a coach who guides you to become the best version of yourself.

Progress tracking and goal adjustment form the backbone of a successful fitness plan. They keep you informed, motivated, and on the right path. Each step teaches you more about your body and what it can do. This knowledge empowers you to make informed decisions about your health and well-being. You keep your fitness routine dynamic and rewarding by consistently tracking your progress and setting new challenges. This approach ensures you continue to grow stronger, healthier, and more confident with every workout.

3.3 SAFETY FIRST: IDENTIFYING WARNING SIGNS

While Therapeutic Exercise is a powerful tool for health and wellness, knowing when to rest is just as important. Exercises come with signs we shouldn't ignore. Sharp or persistent pain is one of them. This kind of pain suggests something is wrong. It's your body's way of telling you to stop and reassess. Unusual fatigue or dizziness during or after exercise is another red flag. This can mean you're pushing too hard or need more rest. It's crucial to pay attention to these signals. They help you avoid injury and overexertion.

If you encounter any of these warning signs, there are steps you can take. Start by stopping the activity and resting. If the pain is mild, gently stretch to ease tight muscles. Ice can reduce swelling if you have a sore spot. For dizziness, sit or lie down until it passes. Drink water to stay hydrated. If symptoms persist, see a doctor. They can help identify the issue and suggest appropriate steps. While it's good to challenge yourself, knowing when to pause is equally essential.

Consulting with a professional is vital. It's common to think you can handle everything on your own. But some situations need an expert's eye. If you experience persistent pain or recurring symptoms, seek medical evaluation. Regular check-ups can catch problems early. They ensure chronic conditions are appropriately managed. Professionals provide guidance on safe exercises and modifications. They help you stay on track without risking your health. Never hesitate to reach out for help when in doubt. It's a sign of strength, not weakness.

Common mistakes can hinder progress. Overtraining is a big one. It happens when you exercise too much without enough rest. This can lead to burnout and injuries. Your body needs time to recover and grow stronger. Plan the rest of the days and listen to your body. Incorrect form and alignment are other pitfalls. Using the wrong form can strain muscles and joints. It reduces the effectiveness of exercises. Always prioritize proper technique over lifting heavier weights or doing more reps. This ensures you get the most out of your workouts safely.

Prevention is key to avoiding these issues. Start by learning the correct techniques for each exercise. If you're unsure, consider working with a trainer. They can teach you the basics and help you build a strong foundation. Gradually increase your workout intensity. Jumping into a high-intensity routine can be tempting, but progressing slowly is better. Your body will adapt and grow stronger over time. Warm up before each session with light movements and stretching. This prepares your muscles and reduces the risk of injury.

Awareness is your most potent tool in ensuring your safety during exercise. It begins with recognizing your body's warning signs and understanding the appropriate responses. Educating yourself on these signals and responding promptly and correctly is paramount to avoiding injury and ensuring your exercises bring wellness rather than harm. Exercise is designed to enhance your well-being, boost your mood, and improve your physical health, not to detract from it. By adopting a mindful and informed approach to your fitness regimen, you can safeguard your health and enjoy the myriad benefits of a balanced and active lifestyle. This proactive stance empowers you to confidently navigate your fitness journey, ensuring that every step you take contributes positively to your goal of achieving and maintaining optimal health.

3.4 EQUIPMENT ESSENTIALS AND ALTERNATIVES

At the heart of any effective exercise program is the right equipment. You don't need a lot, but having a few key items can make a big difference in your workouts. Dumbbells and resistance bands are the foundation for strength training. They're versatile and easy to use. You can adjust the resistance levels, making them suitable for beginners and advanced users. A stability ball is another great addition. It helps with balance exercises and core strengthening. A yoga mat is essential for comfort during floor exercises. It provides a stable surface and prevents slipping. These items create a basic but effective home gym setup. They support a wide range of exercises targeting different body parts.

But what if you don't have access to this equipment? Not to worry. Many household items can serve as substitutes. For instance, water bottles can act as makeshift weights. Fill them with water or sand to add resistance. They are perfect for bicep curls or shoulder presses. Towels can replace resistance bands for stretching and resistance exercises. Roll them up tight and use them to add tension during workouts. You can even use a chair for exercises like tricep dips or step-ups. These alternatives allow you to keep moving without needing to invest in expensive gear. They show that you can maintain a fitness routine with creativity and resourcefulness.

Each piece of equipment brings its benefits. Take kettlebells, for example. They are excellent for dynamic strength training. Kettlebell swings work for multiple muscle groups at once and improve cardiovascular fitness. Foam rollers are also valuable. They help with muscle recovery by releasing tension and increasing blood flow. Using a foam roller regularly can reduce muscle soreness and improve flexibility. These tools enhance your exercise effectiveness, helping you achieve better results. They add variety to your workouts and keep things interesting. They also ensure you work your body differently, which is key to a balanced fitness program.

Selecting quality equipment is essential. You want gear that is durable and safe. When choosing dumbbells or kettlebells, look for a comfortable grip and solid construction. Resistance bands should be made from thick, durable material that doesn't snap easily. For stability balls, check that they are burst-resistant and can support your weight. A good yoga mat should have a non-slip surface and enough cushioning for comfort. Brand reputation is another factor. Brands like Bowflex and TRX have strong reputations for quality. Reading reviews and asking for recommendations can also guide you in making a wise purchase.

Choosing the right equipment is a personal decision. It depends on your space, budget, and workout preferences. Start with the basics and expand as needed. Remember, the goal is to support your fitness journey, not complicate it. Equipment should make workouts more straightforward and practical, not become a barrier. You can take on your personalized exercise program with these essentials and creative alternatives. As you build your routine, you'll find new ways to challenge yourself and keep progressing. This sets the stage for the next chapter, where we'll explore how to incorporate these tools into your daily life.

Step 1: Starting Position

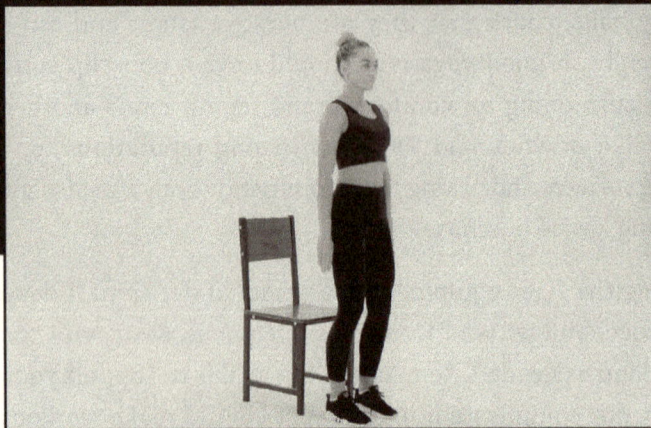

➥ Stand up by pressing through your heels and engaging your core.

Step 2: Perform the Squat

➥ Lower your hips back down toward the chair, keeping your back straight.

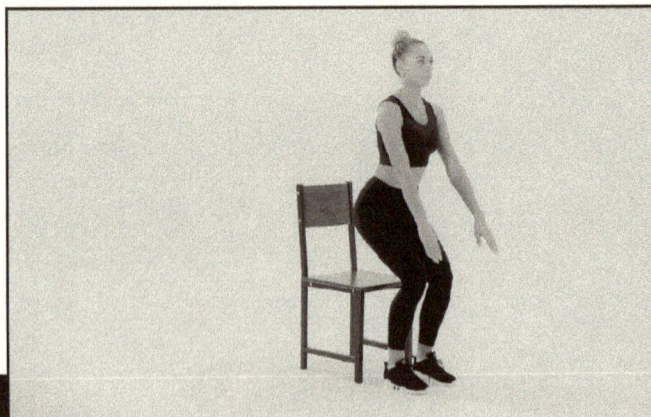

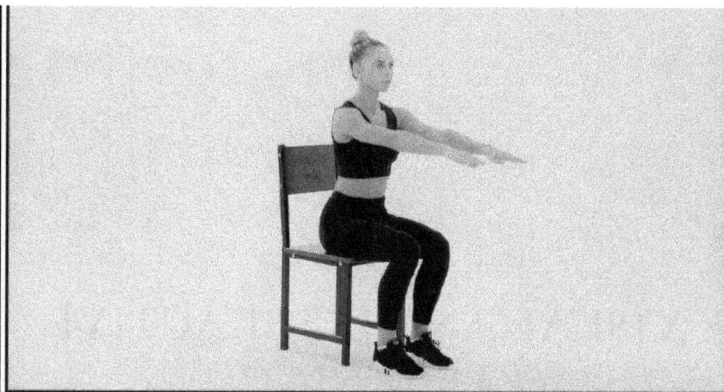

👉 Tap the chair lightly with your hips, then stand back up.

👉 Perform 8-10 reps.

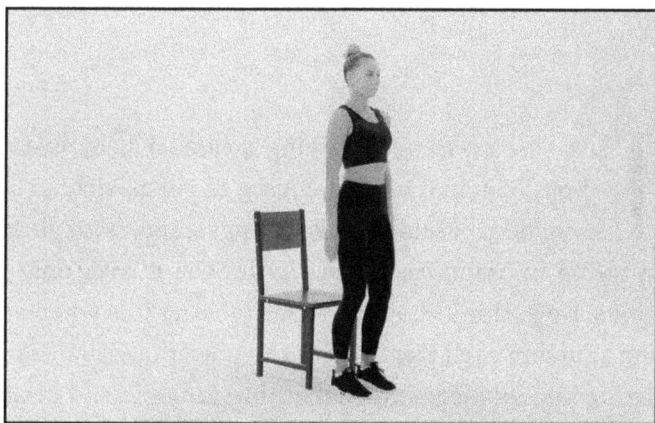

Step 3: Gradual Progression

👉 Start with a few reps and gradually increase the number of squats as strength improves.

4

VISUAL AND INTERACTIVE LEARNING

H ave you ever tried learning a new skill by just reading about it? It can be challenging to grasp without seeing it in action. Visuals make things more straightforward. Imagine trying to assemble a piece of furniture with only written instructions. Now, think about how much easier it is when you have a diagram showing each step. This is the power of visual learning. It transforms complex ideas into something tangible and straightforward. In the world of exercise, visuals can guide you to better form and understanding. They bridge the gap between what you read and what you do. Visual aids help you see your body in a new light. They show you how to move and which muscles to engage. They make the invisible visible.

Diagrams are invaluable in exercise. They provide precise, accurate visual representations to guide proper form and technique. Imagine anatomical diagrams that highlight targeted muscle groups. These visuals show you exactly which muscles you work during each exercise. You can see how your body should look. This guidance helps you perform movements safely and effectively. Step-by-step break-downs take this further. They show each phase of a movement. You see where to start, how to move, and where to end. It's like having a personal trainer in picture form. These breakdowns ensure you know each step of an exercise. They help you avoid common mistakes and maximize your workout benefits.

Visual storytelling takes your understanding even deeper. It narrates the journey of an exercise routine from start to finish. Before-and-after images demonstrate expected outcomes. They show you what you can achieve with consistency. Seeing progress in others inspires you to keep going. Sequential images show how exercises progress. They illustrate how your body can change over time. This visual journey motivates you. It provides a clear path to follow. You see not only where you start but also how far you can go. This storytelling helps you connect the dots between effort and results.

Infographics are another powerful tool. They simplify complex concepts with engaging visuals. Imagine a chart comparing exercise benefits and risks. It lays out information clearly and concisely. You grasp the essentials at a glance. Infographics explaining the biome-chanics of movements are also helpful. They show how your body works during exercise. You see what happens inside your body when you move. This knowledge empowers you to exercise smarter. It helps you understand why proper form matters. It connects the science of exercise with practice. Infographics make learning quick and effective. They turn complicated topics into something digestible.

Interactive Element: Visualization Exercise

Take a moment to visualize your success. Close your eyes and imagine yourself performing your favorite exercise perfectly. Picture each phase of the movement. Feel the muscles working as they should. See yourself reaching your goals. This mental imagery can enhance your physical performance. It prepares your mind for success and reinforces your commitment.

Incorporating these visual elements into your exercise routine enhances your learning experience. They make complex ideas accessible and relatable. Visual aids give you the confidence to try new exercises and refine your technique. They help you see what is possible and motivate you to reach your goals. With these tools, you become both the student and the teacher. You learn about your body and how to move it effectively. Visual learning makes exercise more engaging and enjoyable. It turns every workout into a visual journey of discovery and growth.

4.1 STEP-BY-STEP EXERCISE DEMONSTRATIONS

Getting the steps right in any exercise makes a world of difference. It's like following a recipe. You need to know each part to get the desired result. Start with the initial setup. This is your starting position. It's like the foundation of a house. For a squat, stand with your feet shoulder-width apart. Keep your back straight. Your toes should point slightly outwards. This setup ensures proper alignment and prepares you for the movement. It's crucial to start right to avoid mistakes later on. Next comes the movement execution. Lower your body as if sitting in a chair. Push your hips back while bending your knees. Keep your chest up and your eyes forward. Stop when your thighs are parallel to the ground. This helps prevent strain on your knees.

Resetting for repetitions is just as important. Stand back up by pushing through your heels. Return to the starting position. Take a moment to check your form before going again. This pause allows you to gather your strength and ensure each rep is as good as the first. It keeps your workout effective and safe. Repetition builds muscle memory, making the movement easier and smoother over time. Each squat becomes more natural with practice, improving your balance and strength.

Avoiding common mistakes can save you from injury. Incorrect posture is a frequent error. Many people lean too far forward during squats. This puts extra stress on the lower back. Instead, imagine sitting back in a chair. Keep your weight balanced over your heels. Overextension is another pitfall. Going too low can strain your joints. If you feel discomfort, adjust your range and focus on maintaining control. Using a mirror or recording yourself can help spot these mistakes. Visual cues guide you in correcting them and refining your technique.

Exercises should fit your skill level. Beginners might find full squats challenging. Start with a simplified version. Use a chair for support. Lower yourself until you lightly touch the chair, then return to standing. This helps build confidence and strength gradually. Intermediate users might hold a lightweight device. This adds resistance and increases difficulty. Advanced practitioners can add weight and try deeper squats. Progressions keep you challenged and engaged. They ensure your workouts evolve as you grow stronger.

Safety tips are the backbone of any exercise routine. Proper breathing enhances performance. Inhale as you lower your body. Exhale as you return to standing. This rhythm supports your movement and maintains energy. Joint protection is equally crucial. Keep your knees aligned with your toes to avoid twisting. Warm up before exercising to prepare your muscles and joints. Stretching after a workout helps recovery and flexibility. These habits keep you injury-free and ready for the next session.

4.2 SAFETY REMINDER: CHECK YOUR SURROUNDINGS

Before starting any exercise, check your surroundings. Ensure you have enough space to move freely. Remove any obstacles that could cause harm. This precaution prevents accidents and keeps your focus on the exercise. A safe environment supports a productive workout.

In these demonstrations, the importance of precision cannot be overstated. Each step meticulously builds upon the preceding one, culminating in a fluid and productive routine. Grasping the minutiae of each movement provides you with a commanding grasp over your workout regimen, empowering you to tailor exercises to your unique capabilities and safeguard against potential injuries. Through diligent practice, these meticulously outlined steps will become ingrained, facilitating movement that is both confident and purposeful. This mastery ensures that you are consistently following the most effective path toward achieving your fitness goals, reinforcing the vital role of precision in the successful execution of therapeutic exercises.

Step 1: Starting Position

🔸 Stand with your back flat against a wall, feet shoulder-width apart, about 2 feet away from it.

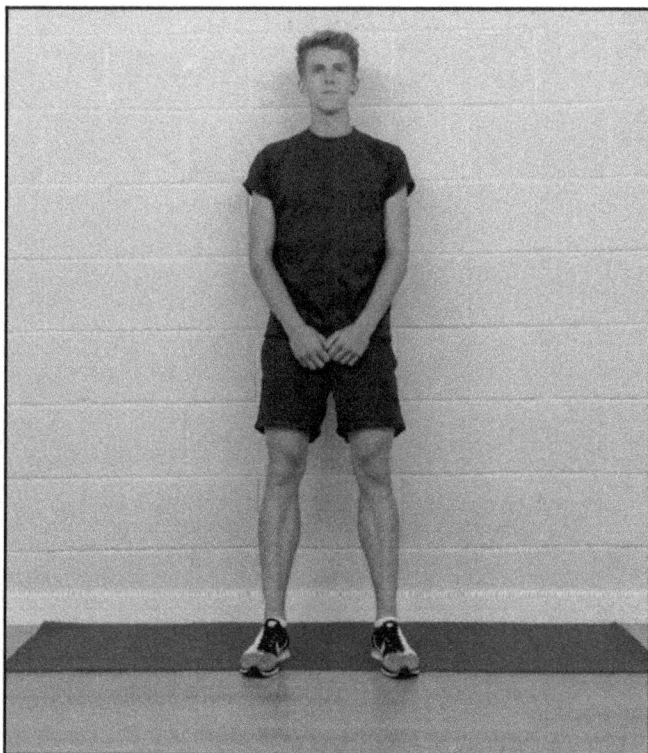

🔸 Engage your core, straighten your spine, and relax your shoulders.

Step 2: Lowering Into Squat

·᠙ᢏᡐ·

🐌 Slowly slide down the wall by bending your knees until your thighs are parallel to the floor.

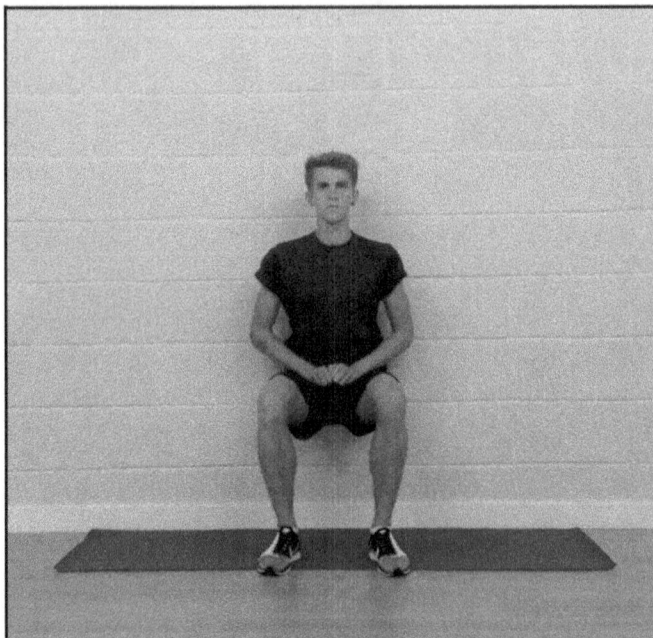

🐌 Ensure your knees do not extend beyond your toes and that your back remains flat against the wall.

Step 3: Mental Imagery

·᠙ᢏᡐ·

🐌 Close your eyes and visualize yourself in a perfect squat, imagining a straight line from your head to your knees.

Focus on breathing deeply, engaging your core, and relaxing your muscles while maintaining the squat.

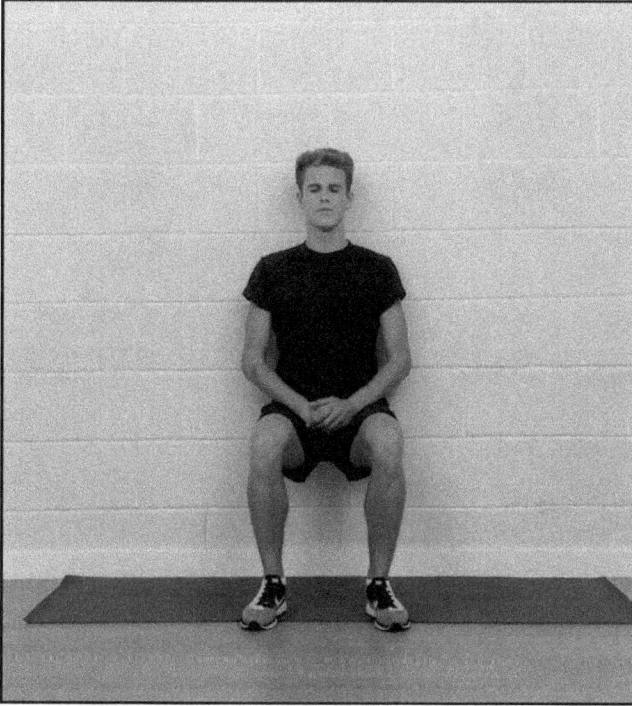

Step 4: Holding the Position

Maintain the squat position, keeping your core engaged and your spine neutral.

Practice deep breathing while holding the position. Focus on mindful alignment with each breath.

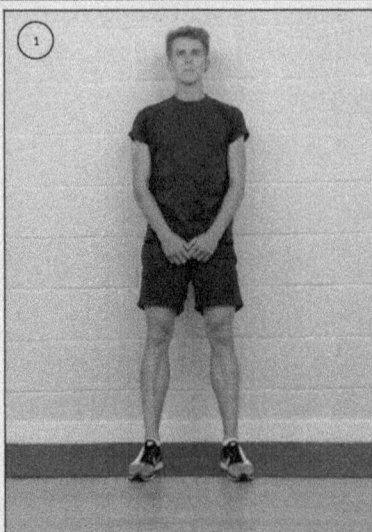

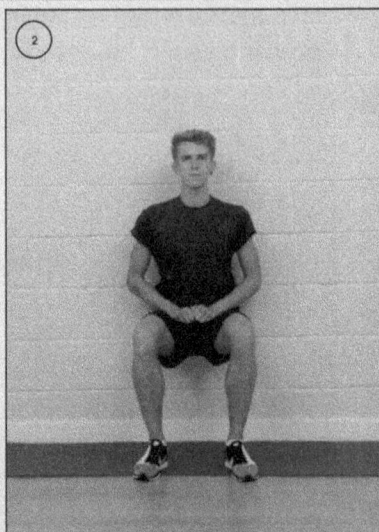

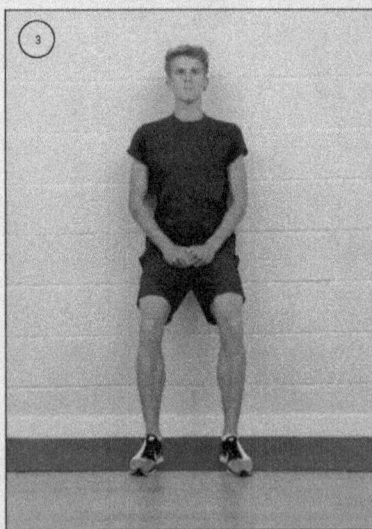

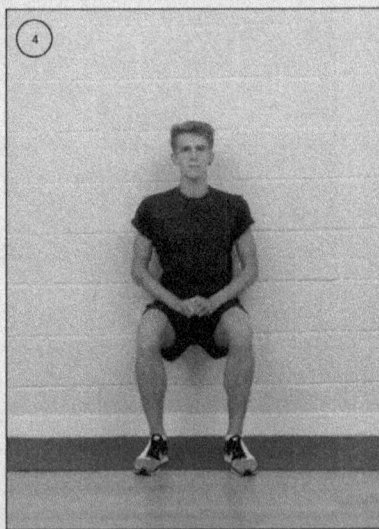

4.3 INTERACTIVE PROGRESS TRACKERS

Staying on track with your workouts can feel like navigating without a map. That's where digital tracking tools come in. They offer a way to log workouts, set milestones, and celebrate achievements. Imagine opening an app and seeing a record of every workout you've done. You spot trends and see improvements over time. This digital log becomes a mirror, reflecting your hard work and dedication. Apps often send notifications when you reach a goal, giving you that extra pat on the back. These reminders keep you motivated, nudging you to push a little more complicated. They provide a sense of accomplishment that fuels your next workout.

For those who prefer the tangible feel of pen and paper, printable tracking templates are a great alternative. You can print weekly and monthly progress charts. They let you map out your workouts, track habits, and see your growth at a glance. These charts are more than just paper. They hold your fitness story. Each mark on the page represents a step towards your goals. Habit trackers are another helpful tool. They help you maintain exercise consistency. Checking off each day you exercise becomes a ritual. It reinforces your commitment and shows you the power of small, regular actions.

Regular updates are the heartbeat of any progress-tracking system. They keep you accountable and focused. Set realistic weekly goals. You could aim to increase your running distance or add a new exercise to your routine. These small targets are stepping stones. They lead to more significant achievements. Celebrating small victories is just as important. Did you manage an extra push-up or run a bit further? Celebrate it. These moments boost your confidence and remind you of your capability. They turn challenges into opportunities for growth. This positive reinforcement keeps you engaged and eager to continue.

Self-assessment is a valuable part of tracking progress. It allows you to reflect on where you are and where you want to go. At regular intervals, ask yourself simple questions. How do you feel about your progress? Are there areas where you want to improve? These reflections provide insights into your journey. They help you adjust your plans and set new goals. Create space for personal notes and reflections. Write down your thoughts and feelings after workouts. This practice offers a glimpse into your mental state. It shows you how exercise affects your mood and outlook. These notes are private conversations with yourself. They offer honesty and clarity, helping you understand your relationship with fitness.

4.4 FEEDBACK MECHANISM: SELF-EVALUATION PROMPT

At the end of each week, take a moment to reflect. Ask yourself: What went well this week? What challenges did I face? What can I do differently next week? Write down your answers. This self-evaluation helps you learn from your experiences. It's a tool for continuous improvement and growth.

Tracking your progress is more than just numbers and charts. It's about understanding yourself and your body. It's about setting goals that inspire you and celebrating the steps you take toward them. Whether you choose digital tools or paper templates, tracking keeps you engaged and motivated. It provides clarity and direction, showing you how far you've come and where you're headed. Each update, each note, adds depth to your fitness story. They remind you of your strength and resilience. They highlight your ability to change and grow. Progress tracking becomes a companion on your fitness path, guiding you with each step.

4.5 USING FEEDBACK FOR CONTINUOUS IMPROVEMENT

Feedback is like a mirror for your exercise routine. It reflects what you're doing well and what needs a little tweak. Constructive feedback helps you refine your technique and improve your results. Imagine you're doing a lunge. A peer or professional might notice your knee is going too far forward. This simple observation can prevent injury and help you build strength in the right muscles. You might have great form until someone points out a minor adjustment. These insights lead to better outcomes. They make your workouts more effective and safe. Self-assessment tools also play a role. They give you a chance to reflect on your progress. Ask yourself: "How did I feel during that workout? What could I do better next time?" These questions help you stay aware and focused on improvement.

Seeking external feedback can seem daunting, but it opens doors to new perspectives. Engaging with experts and peers provides a well-rounded view of your progress. Finding a workout buddy is a great start. This person can offer support and honest feedback. They may point out things you overlook. Together, you challenge each other to improve. Scheduling regular check-ins with a physical therapist is also beneficial. They provide professional insights and help tailor your routine to your needs. They ensure you're on the right track and making safe progress. These interactions enrich your experience. They introduce new ideas and confirm that you're working towards your goals effectively.

Integrating feedback into your routine requires a system. Think of it as an ongoing evaluation. Start by incorporating feedback into your weekly planning. Review what worked and what didn't. Adjust your exercises based on performance reviews. If you're not seeing the results you want, tweak your routine. You may need to increase intensity or focus on different muscle groups. This process of evaluation and adjustment ensures continuous improvement. It keeps your routine dynamic and responsive to your needs. Each week becomes an opportunity to refine and enhance your workouts.

Success stories of feedback-driven growth are inspiring. They show how valuable feedback can be. Consider someone who struggled with running form. After seeking advice, they learned about the importance of foot placement and posture. This feedback transformed their running experience. They ran faster and with less fatigue. Feedback also helped them avoid injuries, allowing them to enjoy running more. Professional guidance can have a similar impact. Testimonials from individuals who achieved significant milestones often highlight the role of expert advice. A personal trainer might suggest a new strength training technique. This small change can lead to substantial gains. These stories remind us that we're not alone in our fitness pursuits. They show that seeking help and listening to feedback can propel us forward.

Feedback is a powerful tool in your fitness arsenal. It keeps you informed and engaged. It helps you see your progress from different angles. By embracing feedback, you open yourself to growth and development. You turn exercise into a learning experience. This chapter highlights the importance of feedback in exercise refinement. It connects your day-to-day actions with long-term goals. It encourages an open mind and a willingness to adapt. Feedback is not just about pointing out flaws. It's about celebrating strengths and building on them. As you continue your fitness journey, remember the power of feedback. Let it guide you to new heights and deeper understanding. In the next chapter, we will explore how to maintain motivation and mindset, which are key elements that keep you moving forward.

Step 1: Starting Position

🕊 Stand with your back flat against a wall, feet about 6 inches away from the wall.

🕊 Press your lower back, upper back, and head against the wall.

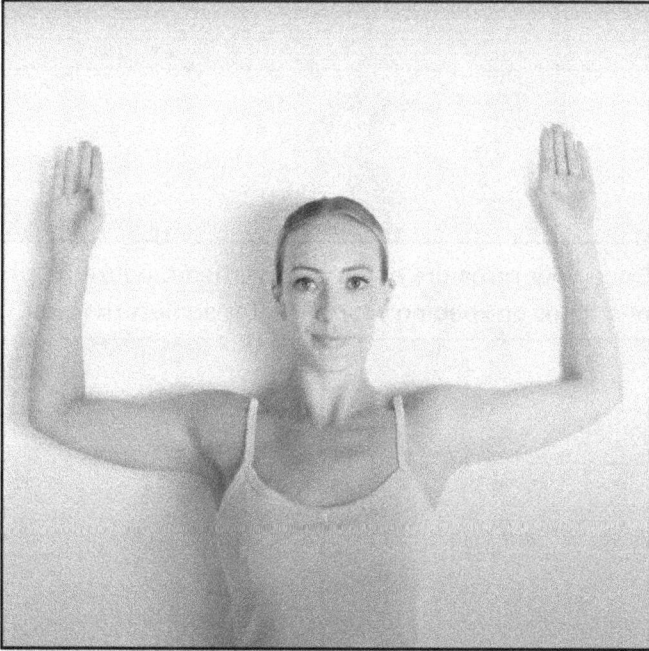

🕊 Raise your arms to a "goalpost" position (elbows bent at 90°), with your forearms parallel to the floor.

🕊 Keep your wrists, elbows, and shoulders in contact with the wall.

Step 2: Perform the Wall Angel

⋙ Slowly slide your arms upward along the wall, keeping your elbows and wrists in contact with the wall.

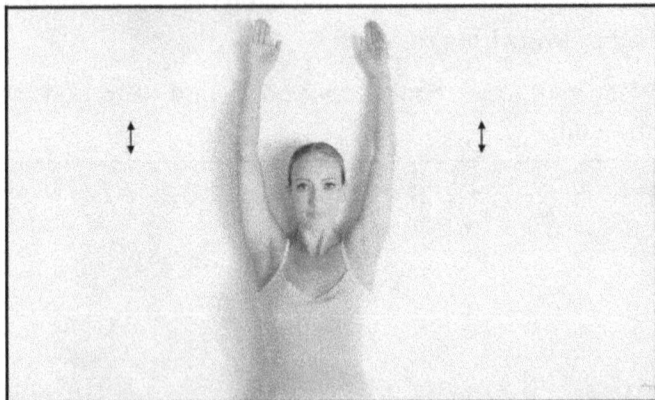

⋙ Once your arms are extended overhead, pause briefly and focus on keeping your back flat against the wall.

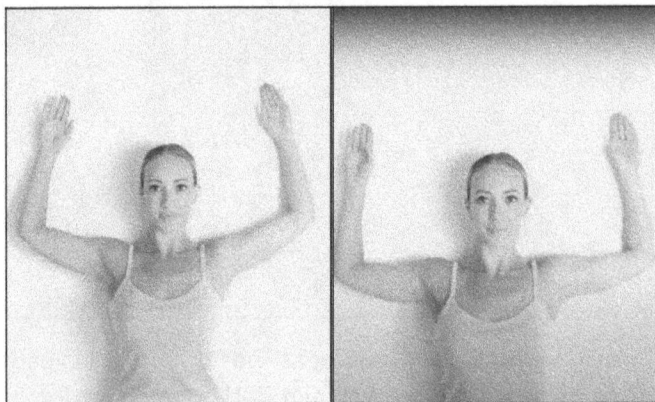

⋙ Slowly lower your arms back to the starting position, maintaining controlled movement.

Step 3: Feedback and Adjustments

꜡ Use a mirror to check your posture, ensuring your back remains flat and your arms move smoothly along the wall.

꜡ If your lower back starts to arch or your arms move away from the wall, adjust your form.

꜡ Perform 10-12 reps, focusing on controlled, slow movements.

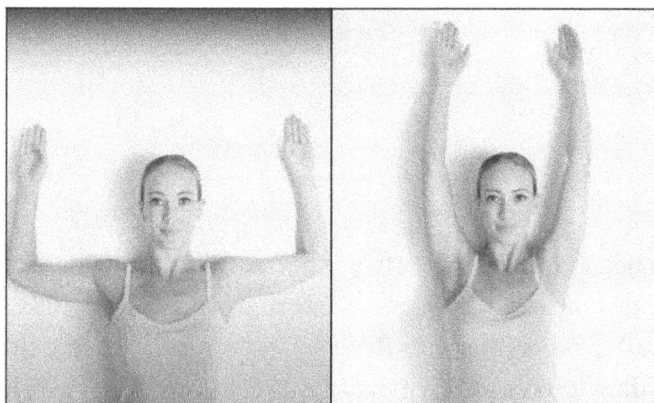

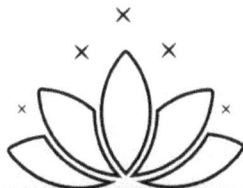

5
REHABILITATION AND RECOVERY STRATEGIES

I magine waking up after knee surgery, feeling hope and uncertainty. You're eager to return to normal activities, but the road to recovery seems daunting. Many people share this experience after knee surgery, whether due to injury or arthritis. The good news is that you can regain strength and mobility with the right exercises and care. This chapter focuses on guiding you through the stages of recovery. We want to help you move from the first days post-surgery to confidently getting back on your feet.

Knee surgery recovery happens in stages. Each stage builds on the last to help you regain full mobility. Right after surgery, you'll start with gentle range of motion exercises. These exercises help reduce stiffness and keep your knee flexible. Imagine doing simple heel slides. Lie on your back, slide your heel toward your body, and then back out. This movement keeps your knee moving without strain. Another early exercise is the straight leg raise. Lie flat, tighten your thigh muscles, and lift your leg. Hold it for a few seconds, then lower it gently. These movements are gentle but essential. They keep your knee from becoming stiff and help with healing.

As you progress to the mid-stage of recovery, you introduce weight-bearing exercises. This is where you start to build strength and stability in your knee. Stationary cycling is an excellent exercise at this stage. It's low-impact and helps improve mobility. Start with short sessions and gradually increase the time as you get stronger. You can also try partial squats. Stand with your feet shoulder-width apart. Slowly bend your knees as if you're sitting back. Keep your weight on your heels and avoid going too low. These exercises strengthen your legs and help your knees support your body weight.

In the late stage of recovery, the focus shifts to strengthening and agility drills. These exercises prepare you for more demanding activities. Step-ups are excellent for building strength. Use a low step or bench. Step up with one foot, then bring the other up to meet it. Step back down and repeat. This exercise targets your thigh and calf muscles. It helps improve balance and coordination. Agility drills, like side steps or gentle hops, add variety and challenge your knees differently. They help improve your reaction time and prepare you for more dynamic movements.

Monitoring your progress is vital throughout recovery. Track weekly improvements in your range of motion. Notice how far you can bend your knee compared to the previous week. Gradually increase the intensity of your exercises. Aim for seven the following week if you start with five minutes of cycling. Write down your progress. It helps you see how far you've come and keeps you motivated. Remember, everyone heals at their own pace. Celebrate small victories along the way.

Precautions and modifications are essential to keep your recovery on track. If you experience swelling, adjust your exercise frequency. It might mean taking an extra rest day or reducing the intensity of your workouts. Listen to your body. Use assistive devices like knee braces if needed. They provide additional support and protect your knee during exercises. Always consult with your healthcare provider before making changes to your routine. They can give personalized advice and ensure you're moving safely and effectively.

Step 1: Starting Position

➥ Lie on your back with your knees bent and feet flat on the floor, hip-width apart.

➥ Keep your arms by your sides and your core engaged.

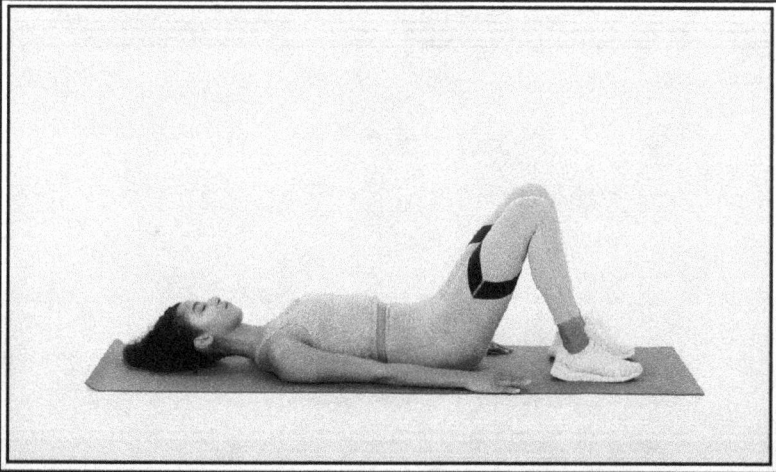

Step 2: Heel Slide

➥ Slowly slide your right foot along the floor, straightening your leg while keeping your foot in contact with the ground.

➥ Return your foot to the starting position, and repeat on the left side.

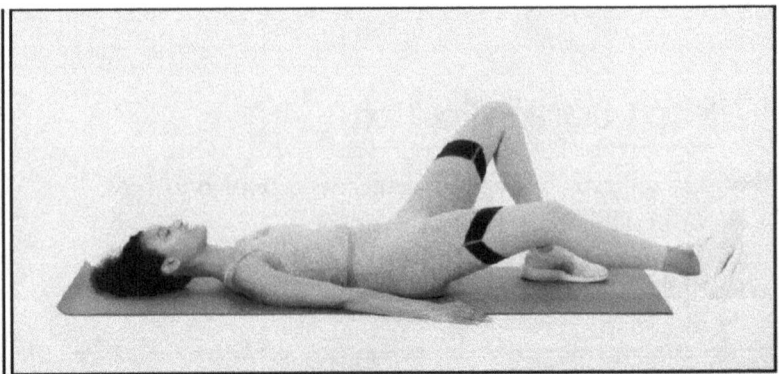
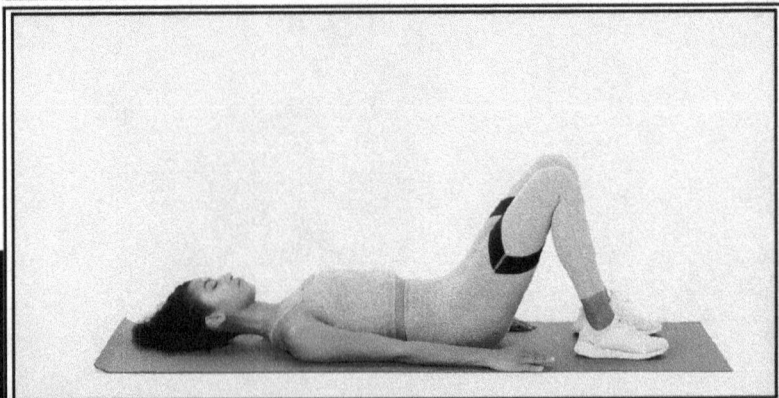
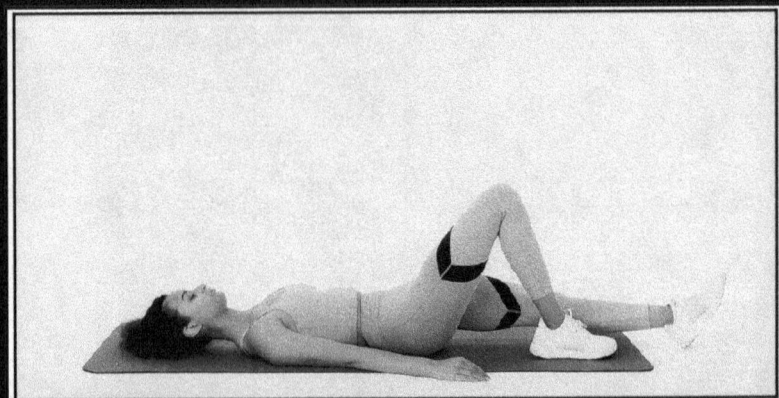

Step 3: Bridge

🐦 Press through your heels to lift your hips off the floor, squeezing your glutes at the top.

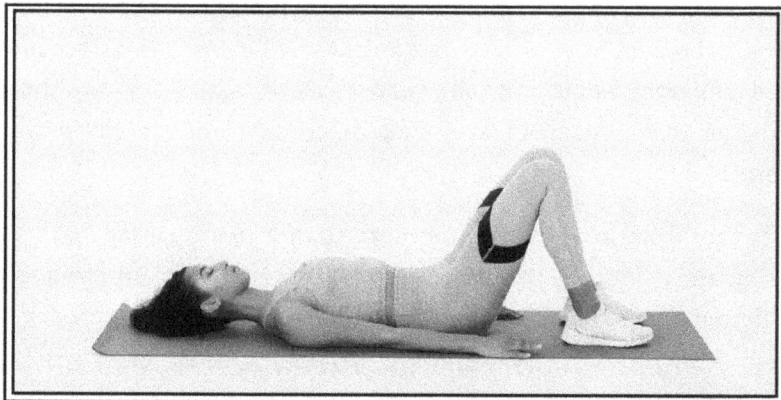

🐦 Keep your shoulders and feet planted while maintaining a straight line from your shoulders to your knees.

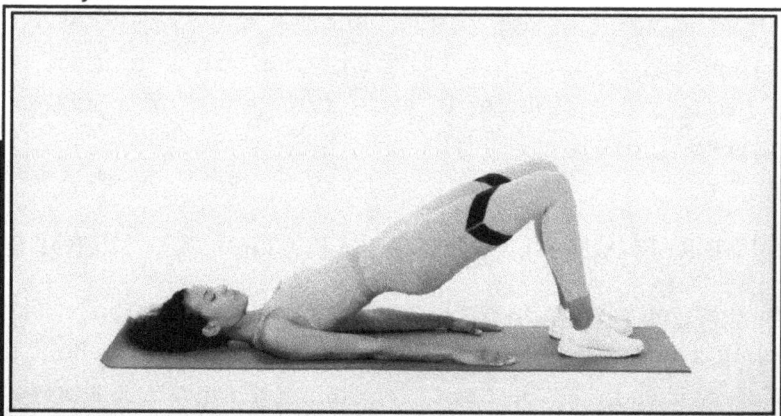

🐦 Hold for a few seconds, then lower your hips back to the floor.

Interactive Element: Progress Tracking Journal

Consider keeping a progress-tracking journal. Write down your exercises, the number of repetitions, and how you feel after each session. Reflect on improvements and setbacks. This journal serves as a personal record of your recovery journey. It helps you stay accountable and motivated. You can also share it with your healthcare provider to get feedback and make necessary adjustments to your plan.

Recovery from knee surgery is more than a mere passage of time; it's an active journey toward reclaiming your mobility and strength. It demands patience, persistence, and a meticulous approach to your rehabilitation. By adhering to the outlined exercises and guidelines, you're not just passively waiting to get better—you're taking decisive, proactive steps toward your healing. Each exercise is a building block towards constructing a knee that's not only recovered but also stronger and more resilient than before. This chapter equips you with the tools and the knowledge to navigate this journey, ensuring that every step you take is informed and deliberate and contributes to your ultimate goal of a successful recovery.

5.1 HIP REPLACEMENT REHABILITATION TECHNIQUES

Imagine you've just had hip replacement surgery. You're likely feeling a mix of anticipation for relief and uncertainty about the recovery ahead. The journey to regaining full function begins with understanding the recovery phases. Initially, rest is crucial. Your body needs time to heal from the surgery. During these first few days, controlled movements are key. Simple actions like ankle pumps keep you active without straining your new hip. These exercises help improve blood flow and prevent stiffness. Another early exercise is the thigh squeeze. Lie down and gently press your knees together. This activates your thigh muscles and supports your healing process.

As you move into the next phase, you focus on enhancing mobility. Standing knee raises become part of your daily routine. Stand up straight, lift one knee comfortably, then lower it back down. This exercise strengthens your hip flexors. Heel-toe walking is another valuable exercise. Stroll, placing one foot directly in front of the other. This movement improves balance and coordination. By incorporating these exercises, you gradually increase your range of motion and build confidence in your new joint. Consistent practice of these movements helps you transition smoothly into the next stage of recovery.

The final phase of recovery emphasizes strengthening and balance. This is where resistance-based exercises come into play. Hip abduction exercises are practical here. Use a resistance band around your legs. Stand with feet hip-width apart. Move one leg to the side, keeping it straight. This exercise targets the muscles around your hip, reinforcing stability. Balance restoration is equally important. Try standing on one leg for a few seconds. This builds the muscles that support your hip and improves your overall balance. These exercises prepare you for more demanding physical activities and help prevent future injuries.

Recovery from hip replacement surgery comes with challenges. Swelling and inflammation are common. It's essential to manage these symptoms to ensure a smooth recovery. Elevate your leg whenever possible and apply ice to reduce swelling. Pain management is also crucial. Modify exercises to reduce discomfort. If a movement causes pain, stop and rest. Gradually reintroduce the exercise at a slower pace. Patience is vital. Recovery takes time, and pushing too hard can lead to setbacks. Listen to your body and adjust your routine to stay on track.

Safety is a priority during hip recovery. Avoid high-impact activities like running or jumping. These movements can put stress on your new joint and hinder your progress. Instead, focus on low-impact exercises that build strength without causing harm. Proper posture is essential during exercises. Keep your back straight and engage your core. This alignment protects your hip and reduces the risk of injury. Always warm up before exercising. Gentle stretching prepares your muscles and joints for activity. Hydration is also essential. Drink plenty of water to keep your body functioning well during recovery.

5.2 SAFETY TIPS: DOS AND DON'TS

To ensure a safe and effective recovery after hip replacement surgery, adhere to the following detailed safety tips: - **Maintain a Regular Exercise Schedule:** Establishing a consistent exercise routine is crucial for steady progress. Set a schedule that includes daily exercises recommended by your healthcare provider. Consistency in your rehabilitation activities helps maintain the momentum of your recovery and can prevent setbacks. **Selecting the Right Supportive Footwear:** When embarking on your journey through therapeutic exercise, one of the foundational steps is choosing footwear that provides exceptional support and stability. Opt for shoes with a well-cushioned sole designed to absorb impact and reduce stress on your joints. The soles should be slip-resistant, offering a firm grip on various surfaces to lower the risk of slips and falls significantly. This is particularly crucial as you work towards regaining mobility, especially after procedures such as hip replacement surgery, where protecting the integrity of your new joint is paramount. Additionally, ensure the footwear has a comfortable fit, with enough room to accommodate any swelling, yet snug enough to prevent unnecessary movement within the shoe that could lead to instability. This combination of cushioning, grip, and fit not only contributes to the safety and effectiveness of your therapeutic exercises but also supports your overall journey towards enhanced movement and well-being.

Listen to Your Body: Pain is an essential indicator from your body that something may be amiss. If you experience discomfort during your exercises, don't dismiss it. Pain beyond mild discomfort could signal overexertion or improper technique. Adjust your activity level accordingly and consult with your healthcare provider if the pain persists. - **Prioritize Controlled Movements:** Rushing through your exercises can compromise their effectiveness and increase the risk of injury. Focus on performing each movement with control and precision. This approach ensures that you engage the correct muscles and avoid placing undue stress on your hip. Taking the time to execute exercises properly supports a safer recovery and builds a stronger foundation for long-term mobility. Incorporating these comprehensive safety measures into your recovery plan promotes a smooth and successful rehabilitation process following hip replacement surgery. By focusing on routine, support, attentive self-care, and precision, you lay the groundwork for a return to your daily activities with confidence and ease.

5.3 SHOULDER SURGERY RECOVERY PROGRAMS

When you face shoulder surgery, the path to recovery can seem long and uncertain. Understanding the phases of shoulder recovery helps you navigate this process with confidence. The first stage involves immobilization and passive movement. This means your shoulder needs time to heal with minimal activity. You might wear a sling to keep your shoulder stable. During this phase, gentle movements like pendulum exercises help maintain mobility without straining your shoulder. Imagine leaning forward, letting your arm hang freely, and drawing small circles with your hand. This simple exercise keeps your shoulder joint from becoming stiff while promoting blood flow and healing.

As your shoulder begins to heal, you begin active movement and strengthening. This stage focuses on regaining control and building stability. Isometric shoulder exercises are key here. These exercises involve contracting your shoulder muscles without moving the joint. For instance, you can press your hand against a wall without moving your arm, engaging your shoulder muscles. This strengthens the muscles and protects the joint. As you progress, resistance band exercises become part of your routine. Using a band, you perform movements like external rotations. This exercise targets specific muscles around your shoulder, enhancing strength and flexibility. Resistance bands offer a safe way to gradually increase intensity without risking injury.

The final stage of shoulder recovery involves functional and sport-specific training. This phase prepares you for daily activities and any sports you enjoy. Exercises mimic real-life movements, helping you regain confidence in your shoulder's abilities. You might practice reaching overhead or lifting objects, gradually increasing the weight as you get stronger. This stage focuses on coordination and endurance, ensuring your shoulder can handle the demands of everyday life. Sport-specific training, for those who play sports, involves drills that replicate their sport's movements. This helps you transition back into your favorite activities with ease and safety.

Gradual progression is crucial throughout shoulder recovery. It's tempting to rush back into activities, but a careful increase in exercise intensity is essential. Monitor your pain levels and range of motion closely. If an exercise causes pain, pause and evaluate. Feeling some discomfort is normal, but sharp pain signals a need to adjust. As you build strength, increase the resistance in your exercises. Start with lighter bands or weights and progress to heavier ones as you improve. This gradual approach ensures your shoulder adapts without strain, reducing the risk of setbacks.

Preventing re-injury is paramount as you work towards regaining full mobility in your shoulder. Initiating every exercise session with proper warm-up techniques is not just beneficial; it's essential. Start by warming up your shoulder with a series of gentle movements and stretches, targeting the muscles around your shoulder girdle. This preparatory step enhances blood flow to the muscles, making them more pliable and less prone to injury. Consider incorporating dynamic stretches that mimic the movements you'll be performing during your main exercise session, as this can further prime your muscles for the activity ahead. In addition to warming up, making ergonomic adjustments to your daily routines can significantly prevent re-injury. Ergonomics—the study of people's efficiency in their working environment—emphasizes the importance of posture and the arrangement of your workspace. When sitting or working at a computer, be mindful of your posture. Ensure that your chair and desk height allow your feet to rest flat on the floor, with your knees and hips at a 90-degree angle. Your computer screen should be at eye level to avoid tilting your head forward or straining your neck, which can indirectly stress your shoulders. Additionally, it's crucial to ensure your shoulders remain relaxed and properly aligned, avoiding a forward hunch or an exaggerated retraction. By optimally positioning your keyboard and mouse so that your elbows stay close to your sides, you can preserve this natural shoulder alignment, effectively minimizing the strain on your shoulder muscles. This adjustment not only aids in maintaining a healthy posture but also significantly contributes to reducing the risk of exacerbating shoulder discomfort or injury. When engaging in activities that require reaching or lifting, especially overhead, take measures to minimize stress on your shoulders. Avoid lifting heavy objects above your head; instead, use step stools or ladders to bring yourself up to the level of the task. When lifting is unavoidable, ensure you use proper techniques—keeping objects close to your core, bending at the knees, and using your legs to lift—to distribute the load more evenly and reduce the load on your shoulders. Implementing these small yet impactful changes in how you approach physical activity and manage your environment can protect your shoulder from re-injury. By incorporating thorough warm-ups, ergonomic principles in your daily activities, and safe lifting techniques, you create a more shoulder-friendly environment, facilitating a smoother recovery and long-term shoulder health. Rehabilitation following shoulder surgery is a nuanced journey of regaining strength and functionality while meticulously avoiding the risks of overexertion. The pathway to recovery is deliberately segmented into progressive stages, each designed to build upon the previous, facilitating a gradual and safe return to your daily routines and activities. Embracing a well-structured rehabilitation plan tailored to your unique circumstances and attentively tuning into the signals your body communicates positions you for a successful recovery. These carefully selected exercises and strategic approaches serve not merely as a roadmap to recovery but as a beacon of empowerment. They instill a sense of confidence, illuminating the path forward and ensuring each step taken in the healing process is informed, purposeful, and conducive to fortifying your shoulder's strength and resilience.

Purpose: These stages outline a progressive recovery plan post-surgery, focusing on restoring movement, rebuilding strength, and returning to functional tasks based on the body's readiness at each phase.

STAGE 1: EARLY STAGE (FOCUS: MOBILITY & CIRCULATION)

Why: Immediately after surgery, the goal is to prevent stiffness, promote blood flow, and initiate light muscle activation with minimal joint stress.

EXAMPLE: ANKLE PUMPS

Step 1: Starting Position

Lie on your back or sit comfortably with your legs extended.

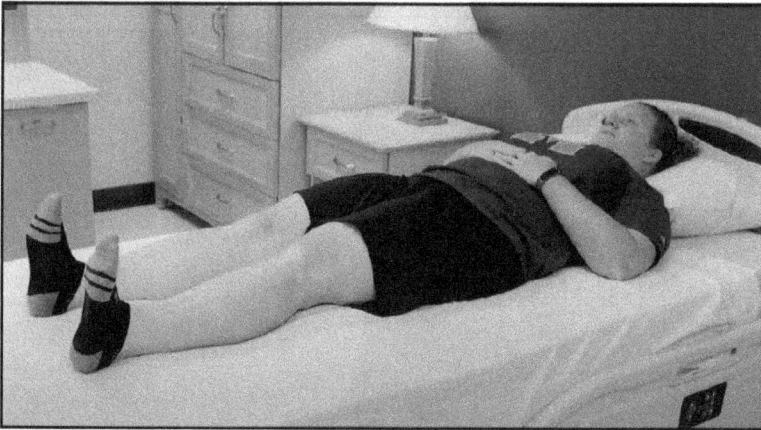

Step 2: Movement

⤷ Gently flex your foot to point your toes upward, then point them downward.

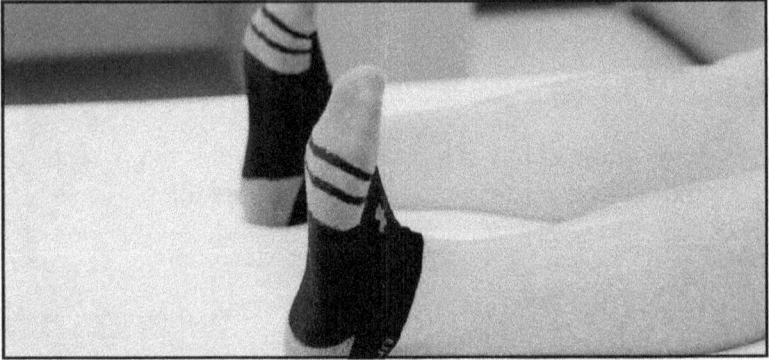

⤷ Repeat this motion slowly and rhythmically for 15–20 reps per foot.

⤷ Perform 2–3 sets per day.

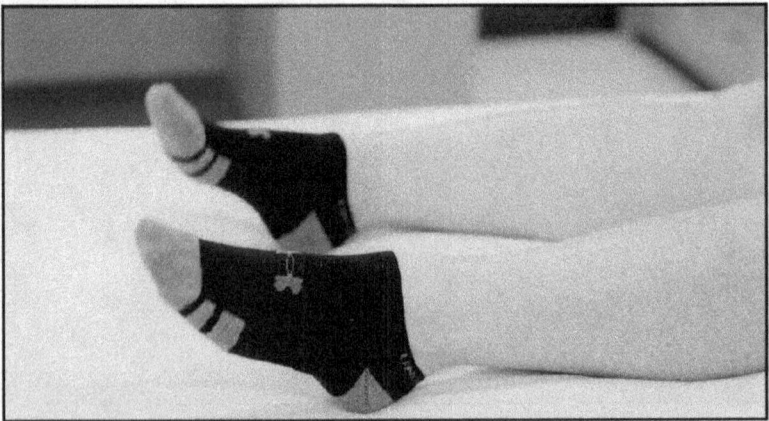

5.4 MANAGING CHRONIC PAIN THROUGH EXERCISE

Chronic pain can feel like a constant shadow, following you throughout your day. It affects millions of adults and can make even the simplest tasks overwhelming. But there is hope. Exercise offers a powerful way to manage and reduce chronic pain. When you exercise, your body releases endorphins. These natural chemicals are your body's painkillers. They help relieve pain and make you feel better. This is why many people notice that their pain decreases after regular physical activity. Exercise also increases flexibility and muscle strength. Stronger muscles support your joints better, reducing strain and discomfort.

Choosing the right exercises is essential. You want activities that are gentle but effective. Swimming is a great option. The water supports your body, reducing stress on your joints. This makes it easier to move without pain. Cycling is another low-impact exercise. It strengthens your legs and improves cardiovascular health. Tai Chi and yoga are excellent for flexibility and relaxation. These practices combine movement with deep breathing. They help reduce tension and promote a sense of calm. You can start with basic poses or movements, gradually increasing in complexity as you become more comfortable. These exercises offer a balanced approach to managing chronic pain.

The mental side of chronic pain is just as important as the physical. Living with pain every day affects your mood and outlook. Mindfulness practices during exercise can help. Focus on your breathing and the sensations in your body as you move. This keeps you present and reduces anxiety. Cognitive-behavioral approaches can also be practical. These techniques teach you to change negative thoughts about pain. For example, instead of thinking, "I can't do this," try, "I'm doing what I can today." This shift in mindset can make a big difference in how you experience pain.

Making exercise a part of your daily life doesn't have to be complicated. Start by setting achievable goals. You can take a short walk every evening or spend ten minutes stretching in the morning. Small goals are easier to stick with and build confidence. Creating a supportive exercise environment helps, too. Find a space in your home where you feel comfortable moving. Keep your exercise gear handy so you can start without delay. If possible, join a class or group. Exercising with others can be motivating and provide a sense of community.

You can integrate exercise into your routine in creative ways. Try doing stretches during TV commercials or taking the stairs instead of the elevator. These small changes add up. Keep track of your progress in a journal. Note how you feel after each session. Over time, you'll see patterns and improvements. This tracking helps you stay motivated and adjust your routine as needed. Remember, consistency is key. Even when the pain is more intense, a gentle walk or some light stretching can help. With time and patience, exercise can become a valuable tool in managing chronic pain.

Why: This phase introduces more active range-of-motion and light resistance to rebuild strength and coordination safely.

EXAMPLE: SEATED KNEE EXTENSION

Step 1: Starting Position

🔖 Sit on a sturdy chair with your feet flat on the floor and knees at 90°.

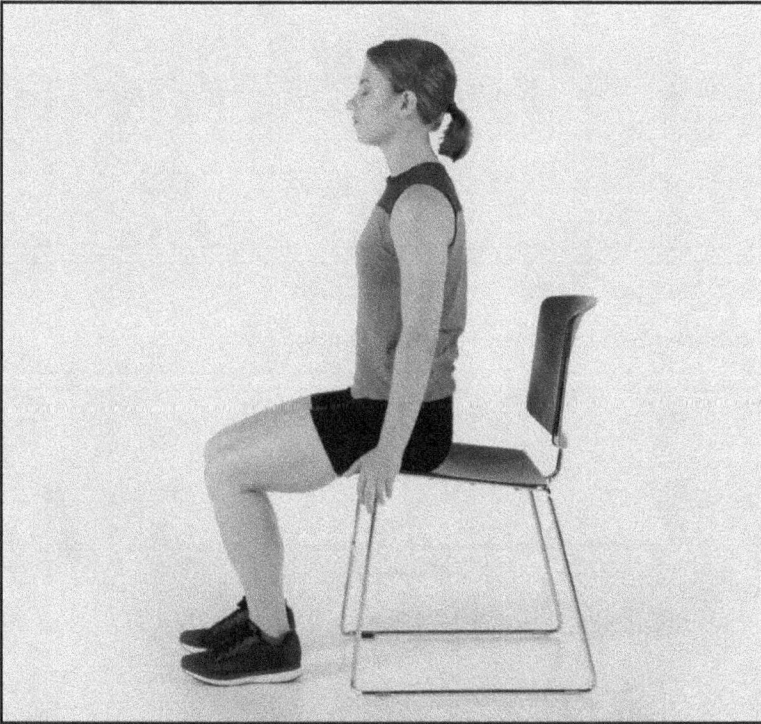

Step 2: Movement

⤳ Slowly straighten one knee, lifting your foot until your leg is parallel to the ground.

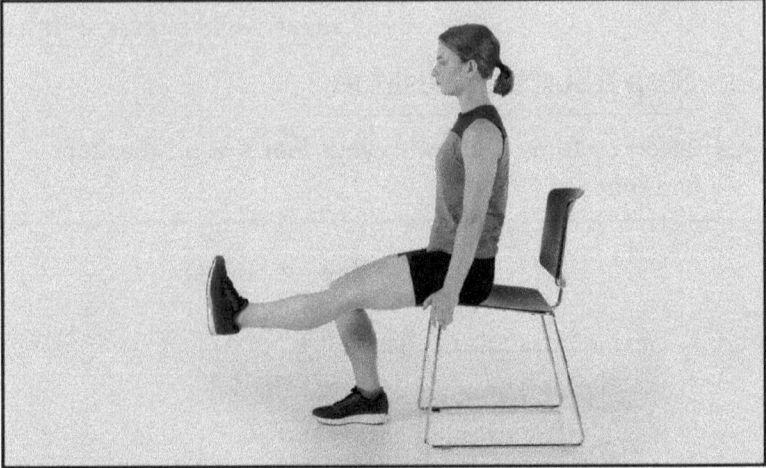

⤳ Pause at the top, then lower slowly.

⤳ Perform 10–12 repetitions per leg.

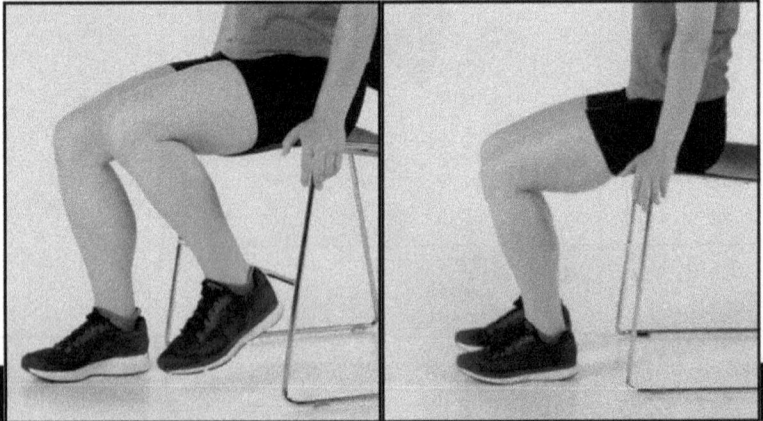

5.5 OVERCOMING FEAR OF RE-INJURY

Facing an injury is challenging, but the fear that lingers afterward can be even more daunting. This fear often centers around the possibility of getting hurt again. Many people worry about feeling that same pain or finding themselves unable to do the activities they love. Anxiety about performance also plays a big part. You might doubt your abilities or feel unsure about pushing your limits. These thoughts are every day, but they can make getting back to exercise harder. It's important to acknowledge these fears. They're a natural part of the healing process. Moving past them requires patience and practice.

Building confidence is key to overcoming these fears. Gradual exposure to exercise can help. Start with activities that challenge you, but do so in a controlled way. Begin with low-intensity exercises that don't stress your body. As you feel more comfortable, slowly increase the difficulty. This approach helps you rebuild trust in your body. It shows you that you can handle more than you might think. Positive reinforcement is also necessary. Celebrate small successes and track your progress. Each achievement, no matter how small, adds to your confidence. Keep a journal of your improvements. Review it when doubts arise. Seeing how far you've come can be a powerful motivator.

Returning to activity should be a phased process. Begin with low-intensity exercises. These allow you to focus on form and control. They help you ease back into movement without overdoing it. Balance and coordination drills are helpful, too. They improve stability and make you more aware of your body. Exercises like standing on one leg or walking heel-to-toe can be practical. They gently challenge your balance and coordination. These drills build a solid foundation for more advanced activities. They reduce the risk of re-injury by improving your body's response to movement.

Professional support plays a crucial role in building confidence. Healthcare professionals like physical therapists, offer guidance and reassurance. They help you create a safe exercise plan tailored to your needs. Regular sessions can track your progress and adjust your program as needed. Support groups are another valuable resource. Sharing experiences with others who've faced similar challenges can be comforting. It reminds you that you're not alone. These groups provide encouragement and practical advice from people who understand what you're going through. They offer a sense of community and support that can be vital in overcoming fear.

Real-life stories of recovery can inspire and motivate you. Consider athletes who've returned to their sport after injury. Their journeys show that it's possible to come back stronger. These individuals faced setbacks and doubts, but they pushed through. Their stories highlight the power of resilience and determination. Athletes often talk about the support they receive from coaches and therapists. They emphasize the importance of patience and gradual progress. These testimonials can encourage you to keep going. They show that overcoming fear is achievable and that success is within reach.

Remember that recovery is a personal process as you work through these fears and rebuild your confidence. It's about finding what works for you and taking it one step at a time. Celebrate each milestone and give yourself credit for your efforts. Overcoming fear takes courage and persistence. Focusing on these strategies and seeking support will pave the way for a safe and triumphant return to activity. Your journey is unique, and every effort you make brings you closer to your goals.

Why: This stage prepares the patient for daily activity and independence, integrating muscle endurance, coordination, and balance.

EXAMPLE: SIT-TO-STAND

Step 1: Starting Position

Sit in a sturdy chair with feet flat, hip-width apart, and arms crossed in front of your chest.

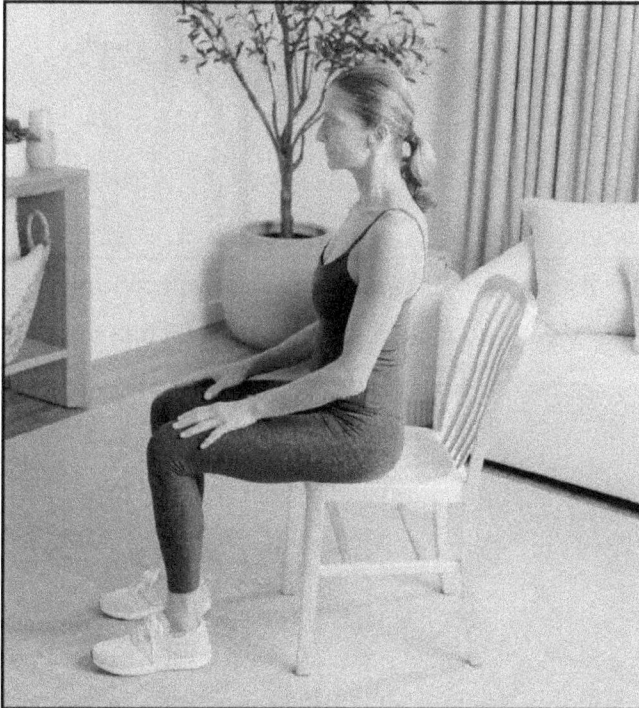

Step 2: Movement

➥ Lean slightly forward and press through your heels to stand upright.

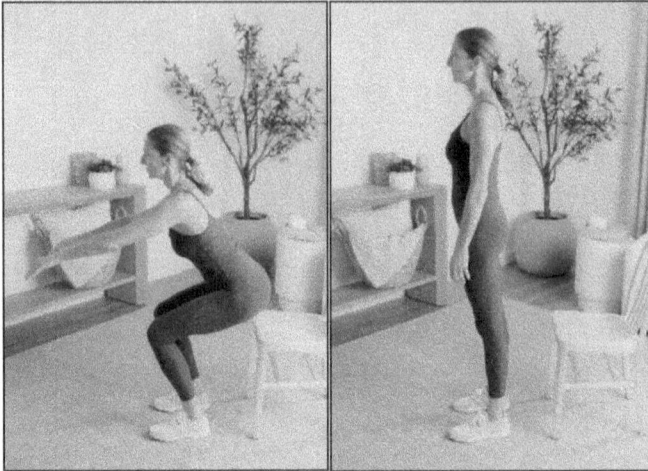

➥ Slowly return to the seated position with control.

➥ Perform 10-15 reps, rest, and repeat for 2-3 sets.

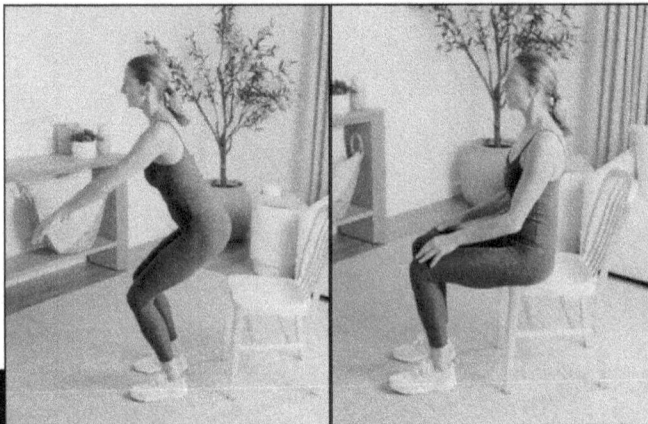

MAKE A DIFFERENCE WITH YOUR REVIEW
UNLOCK THE POWER OF GENEROSITY

"The best way to find yourself is to lose yourself in the service of others."

— MAHATMA GANDHI

Have you ever done something kind just because it felt right? That kind of giving—without expecting anything back—can truly change someone's life.

And today, you have the power to do just that.

Are you someone who once felt stuck—held back by pain, stiffness, or just not knowing where to start with exercise? That's exactly who this book was written for. And there are so many others out there who feel the same way.

That's why I wrote *Therapeutic Exercises Simplified*—to make movement feel doable again. No fancy equipment. No confusing steps. Just easy, clear ways to help your body feel better, one simple move at a time.

But here's the truth: most people don't know where to begin. They scroll, they wonder, they hesitate. And the one thing that helps them decide? **Your review.**

A short, honest review from you can do so much:

- It can guide someone who's nervous about starting.
- It can help them believe that healing is possible.
- It can show them that this book is written for *real people—* just like them.

Writing a review costs nothing. It takes less than a minute. But it can inspire someone to take their first brave step toward a healthier, stronger life.

By leaving a review, you could help:

- One more person get moving again without pain
- One more parent keep up with their kids
- One more grandparent feel steady on their feet
- One more reader feel like they *can* do this

If this book helped you even a little bit, will you help someone else?

☞ Just scan the QR code or click this link to leave your review:

https://www.amazon.com/review/create-review/?ie=UTF8&chan nel=glance-detail&asin=B0FM4MLFZL

Thank you so much for being part of this mission.

With gratitude,

Solomon Cunningham

6

MOTIVATION AND MINDSET

Picture this: you wake up ready to start a new routine, but motivation slips away by the time breakfast is over. You are not alone. Many people struggle with maintaining motivation, especially when goals seem distant. That is why setting the right goals can make all the difference. Well-crafted goals keep you focused and give you a sense of purpose. They act like a compass, guiding you where you want to go. But how do you set goals that stick? One effective method is the SMART framework. SMART stands for Specific, Measurable, Achievable, Relevant, and Time-bound. It transforms vague ideas into precise plans. Instead of saying, "I want to get fit," a SMART goal would be, "I will walk 30 minutes a day, five times a week, for the next month." This goal gives clear steps and a timeline, making it easier to follow.

Short-term and long-term goals serve different purposes. Short-term goals provide quick wins. They boost your confidence and keep you motivated. Think of them as stepping stones. Attending two exercise classes weekly for a month is a good short-term goal. It is specific and achievable. Long-term goals, on the other hand, focus on the bigger picture. They require more time and effort but lead to significant change. Running a 10K by next year is a long-term goal. It requires consistent training and dedication. Balancing short-term and long-term goals keeps you engaged and motivated. It ensures you see progress while working towards more significant achievements.

Personalization is key when setting goals. Everyone's journey is unique. Your goals should reflect your circumstances and aspirations. Personal fitness assessments can help. They show you where you stand and what you need to work on. Consider setting goals that fit your busy lifestyle if you have a busy schedule. You may have a daily commute. Use that time for walking or cycling. If you love being outdoors, set goals that involve hiking or running outside. Aligning your goals with your lifestyle and values makes them more meaningful. This connection increases your commitment and enjoyment.

Tracking your progress is vital for success. It lets you see how far you've come and where to adjust. Digital apps make tracking easy. They log your workouts, monitor your progress, and even remind you of your goals. Many apps offer visual charts showing your achievements at a glance. Regular goal review sessions are helpful, too. Take time each week to assess your progress. Are you on track, or do you need to adjust your approach? These sessions provide an opportunity to celebrate successes and identify areas for improvement.

Setting and achieving goals have psychological benefits. It gives you a sense of direction and purpose. Knowing what you want to achieve helps you focus your efforts. It reduces distractions and keeps you on track. Achieving milestones boosts your confidence. It shows you that you are capable of reaching your goals. Each success builds momentum, making it easier to tackle the next challenge. This positive cycle enhances motivation and keeps you engaged.

Step 1: Starting Position

➤ Stand tall with your feet hip-width apart, arms by your sides, and shoulders relaxed.

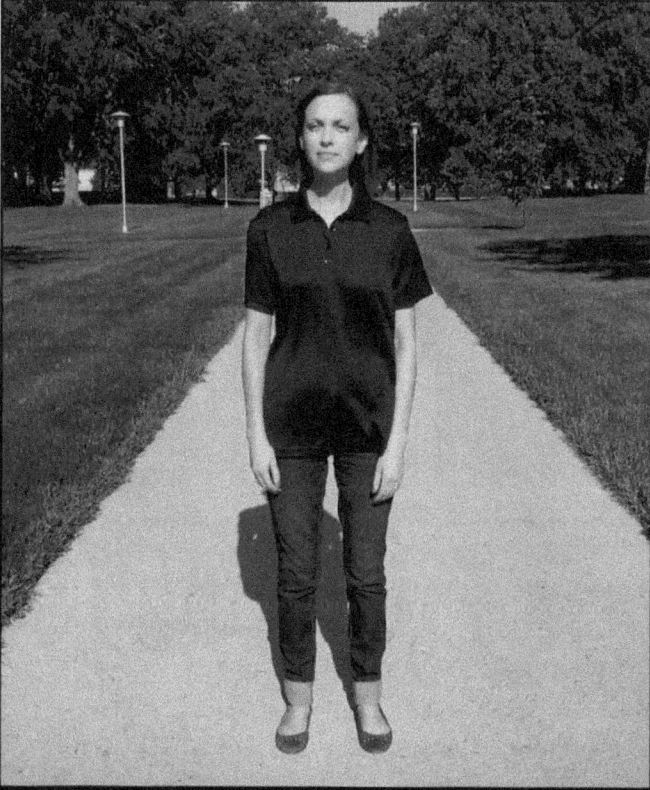

➤ Take a deep breath and focus on setting a clear intention for your walk.

Step 2: Begin Walking

🕊️ Start walking at a moderate pace, focusing on the rhythm of your steps.

🕊️ As you walk, engage your core and keep your posture upright.

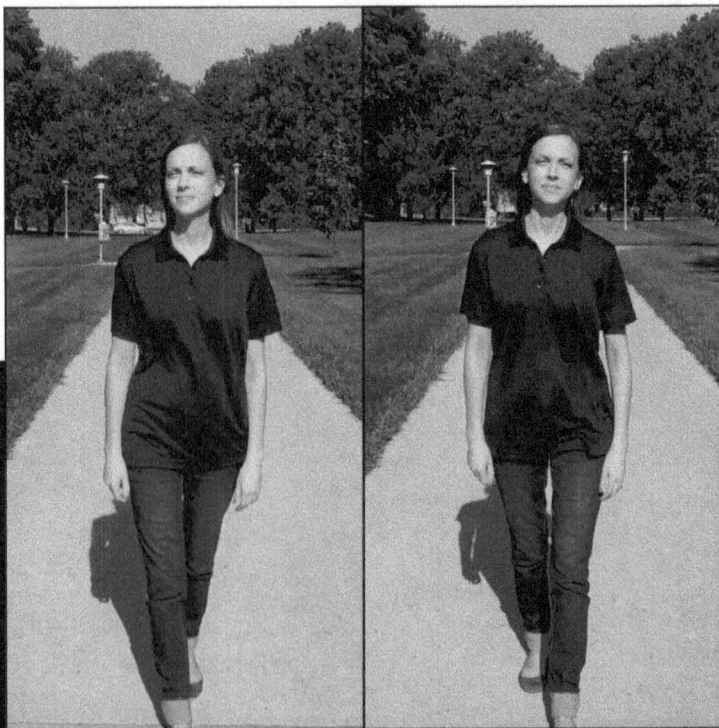

🕊️ Begin walking at a moderate pace, paying attention to each step and maintaining a neutral spine.

Step 3: Focus on Mindfulness

———— ⚬❧⚬ ————

🕊 As you walk, bring your attention to the sensations in your body—how your feet feel as they make contact with the ground, the movement of your legs, and the rhythm of your breath.

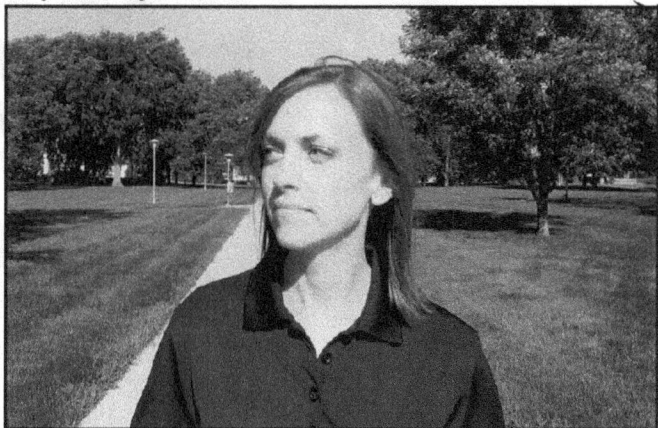

🕊 Pay attention to the environment around you, noticing the sights, sounds, and smells.

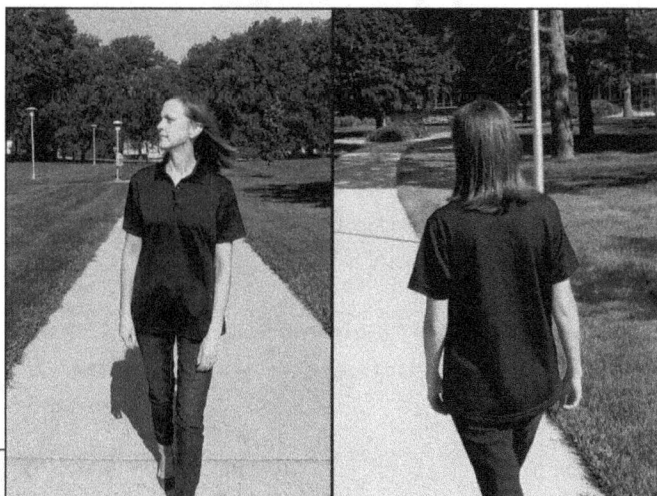

Step 4: Set SMART Goals

➤ **Specific:** Decide on a specific goal for your mindful walk (e.g., walking for 10 minutes or covering a set distance).

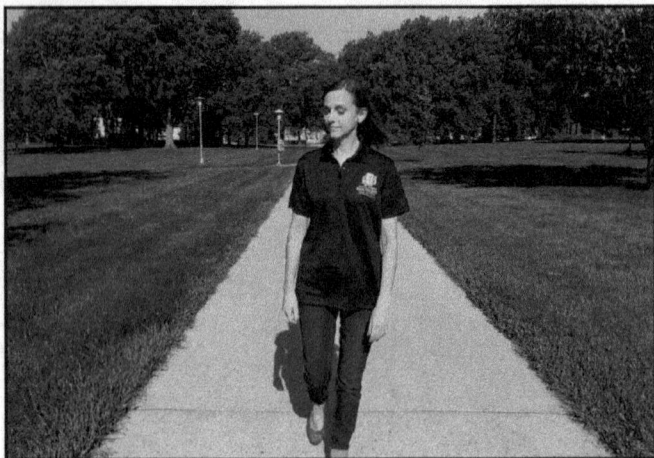

➤ **Measurable:** Track your progress with a timer, step counter, or distance measure.

➤ **Achievable:** Set a goal based on your current fitness level (e.g., walking for 5 minutes if you're just starting).

➤ **Relevant:** Choose a goal that aligns with your broader fitness or wellness objectives (e.g., improving focus, stress relief, or physical endurance).

➤ **Time-Based:** Set a timeframe to complete the goal (e.g., walking for 10 minutes every day for the next week).

Interactive Element: SMART Goal Worksheet

Interactive Element: Crafting Your SMART Goal Plan Dive into creating a detailed SMART goal plan. Start by jotting down your primary goal. Then, meticulously apply each element of the SMART criteria to ensure your goal is well-defined and attainable: 1. **Specific**: Clearly describe your goal. Avoid vague objectives if you aim to improve fitness; specify how. For example, "Increase my stamina by jogging." 2. **Measurable**: Quantify your goal. How will you track your progress? Define this by setting milestones like "Jog for 20 minutes without stopping." 3. **Achievable**: Set a goal that challenges you but remains attainable. Assess your current abilities and resources. Starting with shorter distances might be more realistic if you've never jogged. 4. **Relevant**: Ensure your goal aligns with your broader life aspirations and values. If you value outdoor activities and want to improve your health, jogging outside fits perfectly. 5. **Time-bound**: Establish a deadline. A clear timeframe, such as "Achieve this in three months," gives you a target and helps maintain focus. Break down these elements on your SMART goal worksheet, dedicating a section to each. Reflect on how each part of your goal resonates with your values and fits into your lifestyle. This deep dive ensures your goal isn't just a task on a list but a meaningful step towards a healthier, more joyful life. Regularly revisit your SMART goal plan to monitor your journey. Celebrate milestones, no matter how small, and adjust your plan as needed. This living document is your roadmap, guiding you toward personal growth and success.

By setting achievable goals, you create a roadmap to success. This approach keeps you motivated and focused. It helps you turn aspirations into reality. Remember, the journey is yours. Tailor your goals to fit your life and unlock your potential.

6.1 OVERCOMING COMMON MOTIVATIONAL HURDLES

Life gets busy. Time feels too short. This is a common hurdle that accompanies many who want to exercise regularly. Work, family, and other duties fill your day, leaving little time for anything else. By the time you think about working out, you're tired. It's easy to let your fitness goals slide. But remember, even small pockets of time can work wonders. A ten-minute walk during lunch or a quick stretch before bed makes a difference. The key is to find what fits your schedule. Integrate movement into daily activities. Take the stairs instead of the elevator, or park further away to add more steps. These little changes add up and help you stay active without needing extra hours in the day.

Another challenge is not seeing immediate results. This can be frustrating. You start with excitement, but you lose steam when changes don't appear quickly. It's important to understand that progress takes time. Fitness is not a sprint. It's a marathon. Your body needs time to adapt and grow stronger. Instead of focusing on the result, enjoy the process. Celebrate small victories like feeling more energetic or sleeping better. Reframe setbacks as learning opportunities. If a workout feels tough, see it as a chance to grow. If you miss a session, use it to plan better next time. These moments are part of the journey.

Intrinsic motivation plays a crucial role in staying committed to your fitness goals. Finding what truly drives you can make all the difference. Connect your exercise routine to personal values and joys. If you love nature, take your workouts outside. If you enjoy music, create a playlist that energizes you during exercise. These personal connections transform exercise from a chore into something you look forward to. Journaling can also help. Reflect on your progress and achievements. Write about how exercise makes you feel. Over time, you'll see growth and build a stronger connection to your goals.

Real-life stories offer powerful inspiration. Consider Mary, a busy mom who struggled to find time for herself. She felt discouraged by her slow progress. But Mary started using early mornings for short workouts at home. She found joy in those quiet moments before the house woke up. Over time, her strength grew, and so did her confidence. Then there's Tom, who hit a plateau in his weight loss journey. Instead of giving up, he tried new activities like cycling and swimming. These changes reignited his passion for fitness. He discovered new strengths and kept moving forward. These stories show how persistence and creativity help overcome motivational slumps.

Reflection Exercise: Personal Motivation Journal

Pause for a moment to deeply consider your driving forces. Document the reasons behind your desire to maintain an active lifestyle. Detail the aspects of exercise that bring you joy and outline the emotional and physical sensations you experience during and after a workout. This personal narrative becomes a beacon during dwindling motivation, a powerful reminder of your intrinsic motivation and the personal fulfillment that comes from staying active. Reflect on this journal entry whenever you need to reignite your passion for movement, allowing it to guide you back to your core reasons for pursuing a healthier, more active life.

Facing obstacles is an inherent aspect of our lives, serving as challenges and catalysts for personal growth and resilience. By adopting effective time management strategies and adopting a mindset that values the journey as much as the destination, you can sustain high motivation. It's crucial to remember that progress in therapeutic exercise, like in life, often comes in small increments. Each modest step forward is a victory in its own right, deserving of recognition and celebration. Acknowledging and valuing these efforts, you continuously fuel your journey forward, navigating through challenges with perseverance and a positive outlook. The Power of Accountability Partners

Imagine starting a new exercise routine with a friend by your side. They cheer you on when you feel like giving up. They celebrate your wins and help pick you up after a fall. This support is the magic of accountability partnerships. These partnerships can transform your fitness experience. They bring an extra layer of commitment that's hard to achieve on your own. When you know someone is counting on you, skipping that workout becomes more complicated. This kind of partnership isn't limited to friends. Family members, coworkers, or even coaches can fill this role. The key is finding someone who understands your goals and shares your dedication. A good partner encourages you and keeps you focused. They hold you accountable in a supportive way and celebrate your achievements. This partnership adds a social element to your fitness routine, making it more enjoyable and less of a chore.

Selecting the right accountability partner is essential. Not everyone will suit your needs or schedule. Look for someone who shares similar goals and commitments. You want someone reliable who will stick to the plan. Communication is key, so choose a partner you feel comfortable talking to. Setting clear expectations and boundaries can prevent misunderstandings. Discuss how often you'll meet or check in. You may prefer daily text messages or weekly phone calls. Decide together what works best. Establishing these guidelines early on helps maintain a healthy partnership. It also ensures that both of you are on the same page and ready to support each other effectively.

Keeping the partnership active requires effort from both sides. Regular check-ins are crucial. Schedule calls or meetings to discuss your progress. Share your challenges and brainstorm solutions together. This keeps both of you motivated and on track. Social media can also be a helpful tool. Create a private group to share updates and encouragement. Post about your workouts and celebrate milestones together. This adds a layer of accountability and motivation. It also allows you to connect with others on a similar path. Engaging with a broader community can offer new insights and inspiration.

Being part of a fitness community can amplify your motivation. Joining local fitness groups or online forums connects you with like-minded individuals. These communities offer support and encouragement. They provide a space to share experiences and learn from others. Participating in group challenges or events adds excitement and variety. These challenges push you to try new things and step out of your comfort zone. They also create opportunities to make new friends and expand your support network. Having people who understand and share your goals can make the journey more enjoyable and rewarding.

Interactive Element: Accountability Partner Checklist

Use this checklist to find the perfect accountability partner. Make sure they share similar fitness goals. Ensure they have a compatible schedule and communication style. Discuss expectations and boundaries together. Decide on regular check-in times and preferred methods. Be open to adjustments as needed.

The power of accountability partnerships lies in the connection they create. They offer a unique blend of motivation, support, and camaraderie. Whether it's a friend, family member, or group, these partnerships can keep you on track and push you further than you might go alone. They remind you that you're not in this alone and that someone is cheering for your success.

6.2 CELEBRATING MILESTONES AND ACHIEVEMENTS

Remember the last time you reached a goal, no matter how small. Remember how good it felt? Celebrating these wins boosts your morale and fuels your motivation. These moments are not just lovely —they are powerful. Recognizing achievements, even tiny ones, creates a positive cycle. It shows you that your efforts are paying off.

This positive reinforcement encourages you to keep going. It builds confidence and makes you more likely to tackle the next challenge. When you celebrate, you acknowledge your hard work. You tell yourself you are capable. This mindset is crucial for lasting change.

Creative ways to celebrate can make reaching goals even more rewarding. You don't need to wait for significant milestones. Small wins deserve recognition, too. Reward yourself with something meaningful. It could be a new fitness class you've wanted to try. It may be a piece of gear that makes your workouts more enjoyable. These rewards serve as reminders of how far you've come. Another idea is to host a virtual celebration with your accountability partners. Share your achievements and cheer each other on. This not only strengthens your commitment but also builds community. Celebrations create a sense of accomplishment and make your hard work feel worthwhile.

Reflecting on your progress is an integral part of the celebration. It helps you see how far you've come and what you've accomplished. Journaling exercises are a great way to do this. Write about your journey, noting challenges and victories. This practice offers insight and clarity. It helps you set future goals and plan your next steps. Another creative option is to create a visual progress timeline or scrapbook. Collect photos, quotes, and mementos that represent your achievements. This visual reminder keeps you motivated and focused. It shows you that progress is real and ongoing. Reflection deepens your understanding of what works for you and what doesn't.

Self-compassion plays a significant role in how you celebrate. It's about being kind to yourself through the process. Practicing gratitude and self-acknowledgment enhances motivation. Recognize your effort in each step, even if progress is slow. Avoid self-criticism and perfectionism. They can steal joy and diminish your achievements. Instead, focus on what you've done well. Celebrate every step forward, no matter how small. This kindness fosters a positive mindset. It keeps you engaged and eager to continue. Remember, the path to success is not always straight. There will be bumps along the way. Embrace them as part of your story.

Reflection Section: Gratitude and Progress Journal

Take a moment to acknowledge your hard work. Write down three things you're grateful for in your fitness journey. Reflect on your progress and note one area where you've grown. Use this journal as a tool for self-compassion and motivation.

Celebrating achievements, both big and small, is vital. It builds confidence and keeps your motivation high. By rewarding yourself and reflecting on your progress, you create a positive cycle that encourages continued effort and growth. Embrace self-compassion and gratitude as part of your celebrations. They remind you of your strengths and help you stay on track.

6.3 MINDFULNESS AND STRESS MANAGEMENT

Imagine stepping into a workout with a clear mind, ready to focus on each movement. Mindfulness can turn this image into reality. By bringing attention to the present, mindfulness enhances your exercise experience. Breathing exercises are a simple way to start. Before a workout, take a few moments to breathe deeply. Inhale slowly through your nose and exhale through your mouth. This simple act calms your mind and prepares your body. It lets you focus on your workout without distractions and stress. Another technique is body scan meditation. Lie down or sit comfortably. Close your eyes and focus on each body part, from head to toe. Notice any tension or discomfort. This practice increases body awareness and helps you connect with how you feel. These mindfulness techniques support a focused and fulfilling exercise session, making each movement more intentional and effective.

Managing stress is crucial for maintaining motivation and focus. Stress can drain your energy and make staying committed to your goals challenging. Progressive muscle relaxation is a powerful tool to combat stress. This technique involves tensing and then relaxing each muscle group. Start with your toes and work your way up to your head. It releases tension and relaxes your body. Yoga and Tai Chi are also excellent stress management strategies. They combine movement with breath, promoting relaxation and flexibility. These practices help you find balance and calm in your routine. They teach you to listen to your body and respond with care. Incorporating these techniques into your routine helps reduce stress and enhance your overall well-being.

Exercise itself is a powerful way to manage stress. When you move, your brain releases endorphins. These chemicals boost your mood and create feelings of happiness. They act like natural stress relievers. Regular exercise also improves sleep quality. When you sleep better, you feel more rested and less stressed. This cycle of exercise, endorphin release, and better sleep creates a positive feedback loop. It supports mental and emotional health. By keeping your body active, you reduce stress and enhance relaxation. Exercise becomes a tool for managing life's challenges and fostering a sense of calm.

Mindfulness extends beyond exercise. It can become a part of your daily life, helping you manage stress in all areas. Start by practicing mindful eating. Pay attention to the flavors, textures, and smells of your food. Eat slowly and savor each bite. This practice helps you develop a healthy relationship with food. It also reduces overeating and improves digestion. Daily gratitude journaling is another way to cultivate mindfulness. Each day, write down three things you're grateful for. This simple act shifts your focus to the positive aspects of your life. It increases happiness and reduces stress. These mindfulness practices help you stay centered and present, even in stressful times.

Step 1: Starting Position

🕊️ Sit or lie down in a comfortable position, ensuring your body is fully relaxed.

🕊️ Close your eyes and take a few deep breaths, inhaling slowly through your nose and exhaling through your mouth.

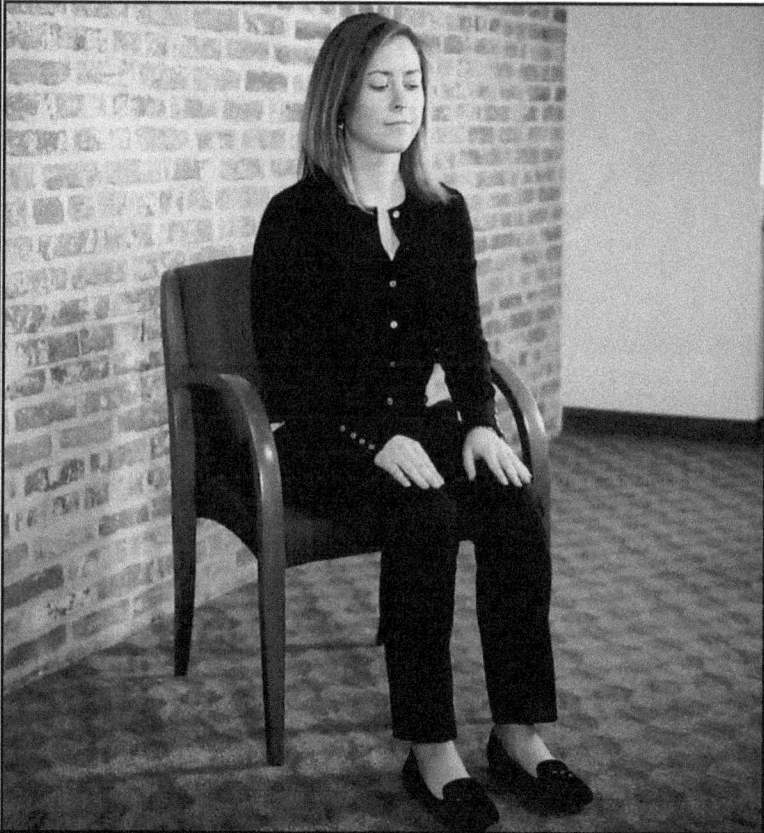

Step 2: Focus on Muscle Groups

—⸳❧⸳—

➥ Begin by focusing on your feet and toes. Tense the muscles as tightly as possible for 5-10 seconds, then release the tension and relax.

➥ Move up the body to your calves, thighs, abdomen, chest, arms, and face, tensing and relaxing each muscle group for 5-10 seconds.

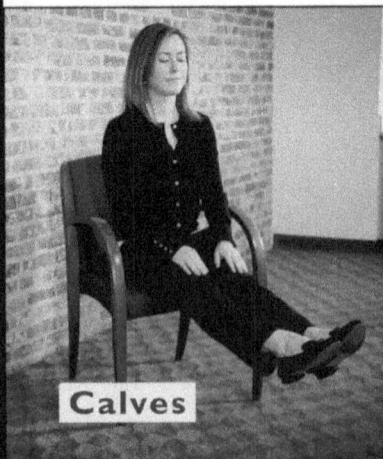

Calves

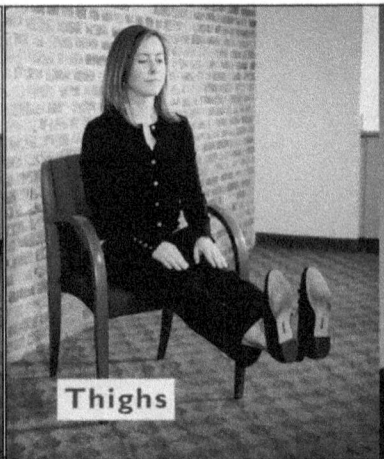

Thighs

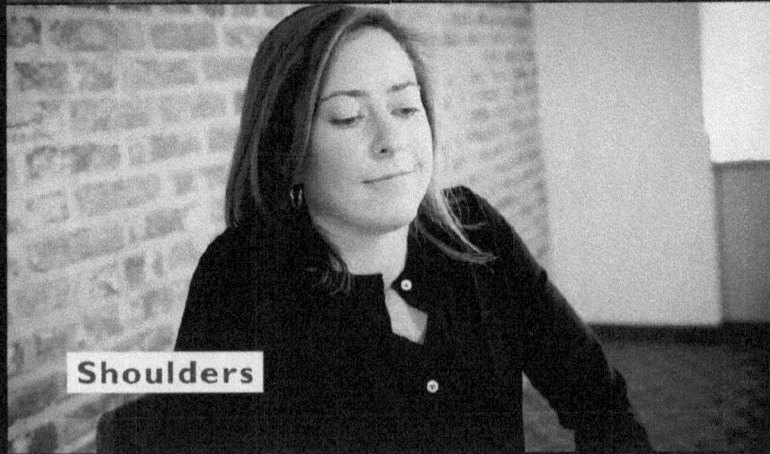

Shoulders

🕊 Pay close attention to the feeling of relaxation after releasing tension in each area.

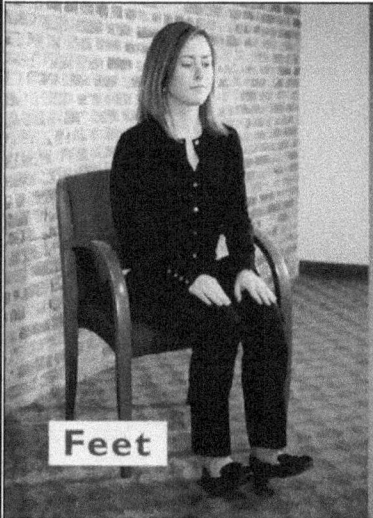

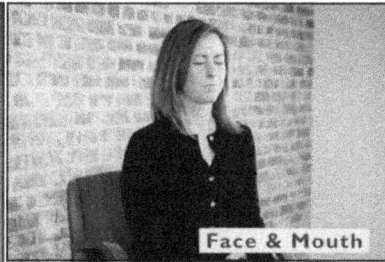

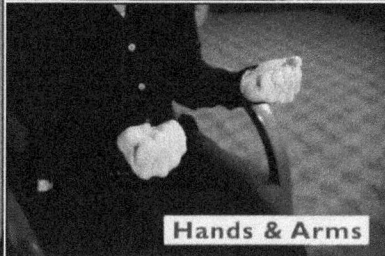

Feet

Face & Mouth

Hands & Arms

🕊 Continue tensing and relaxing each muscle group from your feet to your head, focusing on the contrast between tension and relaxation.

Step 3: Deep Breathing

🕊 After completing the muscle groups, focus on deep, rhythmic breathing. Inhale for a count of 4, hold for 4, and exhale for 4.

🕊 Repeat for 3-5 minutes, focusing on the calming effects of your breath and relaxation.

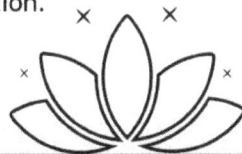

By integrating mindfulness into your routine, you enhance both your physical and mental well-being. It transforms exercise from a task

into a rewarding experience. Mindfulness helps you focus on each movement, making your workouts more effective. It also reduces stress, improving your mood and energy levels. As you bring mindfulness into your daily life, you create a foundation for happiness and health. This approach encourages a more balanced and fulfilling life. With mindfulness as a guide, you effortlessly navigate life's challenges, staying focused and resilient. In the next chapter, we will explore advanced techniques to enhance your exercise routine and well-being further.

7
ADVANCED TECHNIQUES FOR ENHANCED RESULTS

———

I magine you're about to run a race. You wouldn't just jump right in without getting your body ready, would you? Dynamic stretching is like the warm-up lap for your muscles. It gets your blood moving. Unlike static stretching, which is more about holding a pose, it prepares your body for action. Dynamic stretches focus on movement. They increase flexibility and blood flow, making your muscles ready for exercise. Arm circles and leg swings are examples. They wake up your arms and legs, preparing them to work hard. Walking lunges with a twist stretch your legs while also engaging your core. These movements are simple, but they prepare your body for more intense activity.

Dynamic warm-ups are crucial for enhancing performance. They reduce the risk of injury by preparing your muscles and joints. High knees and butt kicks are great for getting your heart rate up. They activate your cardiovascular system, ensuring your body is ready for the workout. Inchworms are another effective exercise. They stretch your entire body. Start standing, bend forward, and walk your hands out to a plank. Then, walk your feet up to meet your hands. This not only stretches your muscles but also engages your core. The world's most excellent stretch combines lunges with a twist, targeting multiple muscle groups. It's one of the best ways to prepare your body for a full-body workout.

Dynamic stretching plays a unique role in different sports. Leg swings and high knees help runners prepare their legs for the repetitive running motion. Cyclists benefit from dynamic stretches that focus on their hips and hamstrings. These stretches ensure their legs can pedal smoothly and powerfully. Team sports like soccer and basketball require tailored routines. Players need to be agile and quick. Dynamic stretches that mimic game movements, like side shuffles and jogging, are ideal. These exercises prepare athletes for the sudden changes in direction and speed needed during a game. Using sport-specific dynamic stretches helps improve performance and reduces the risk of injuries.

Follow a few simple guidelines to incorporate dynamic stretching into your routine. Timing is key. Start your dynamic warm-up about five to ten minutes before your main workout. This allows your body to transition from rest to active mode. Keep the movements controlled and focus on quality, not speed. Aim for about 10 to 12 repetitions for each exercise. This ensures your muscles have enough time to warm up without becoming fatigued. You can move from general stretches to more sport-specific ones as you progress. For instance, a runner might start with high knees and gradually progress to more complex drills like bounding.

Step 1: Starting Position (Inchworm)

🔽 Stand with your feet shoulder-width apart and your arms at your sides

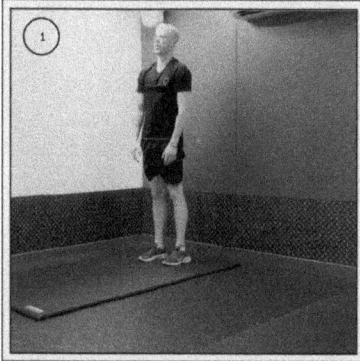

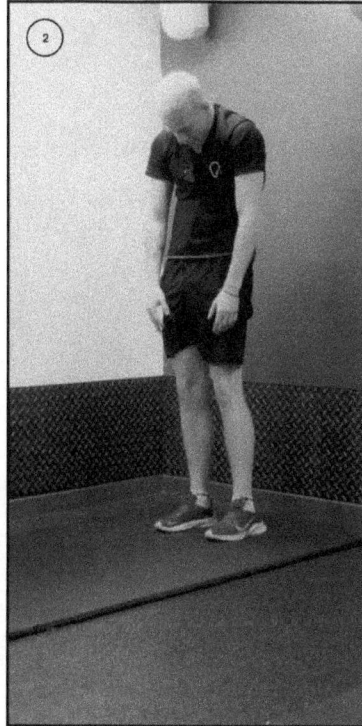

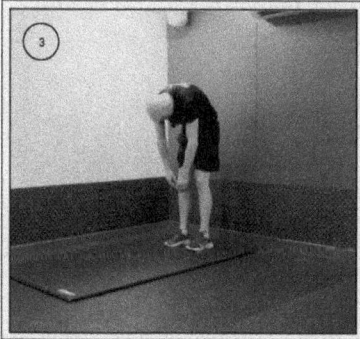

Step 2: Walk Hands Out

🔽 Bend forward at the hips and walk your hands out into a plank position.

🔽 Keep your body aligned, with your core engaged.

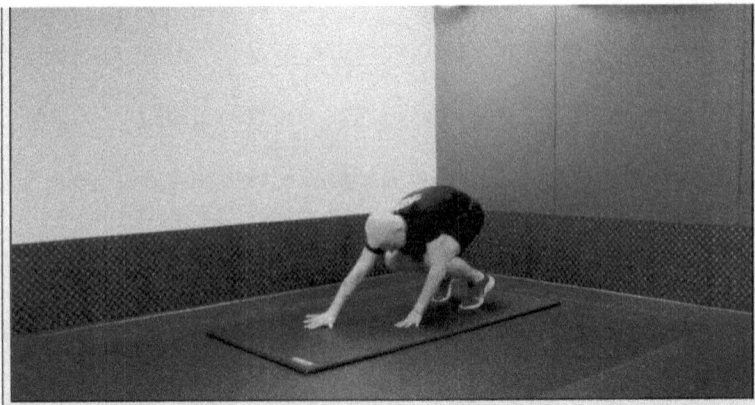

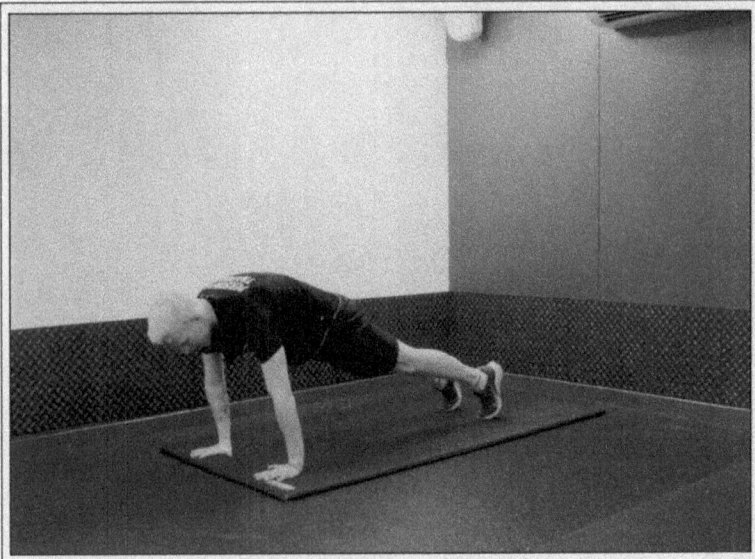

Step 3: Walk Feet In
————————•⟨♋⟩•————————

🢒 Walk your feet toward your hands, keeping your legs straight but not locked.

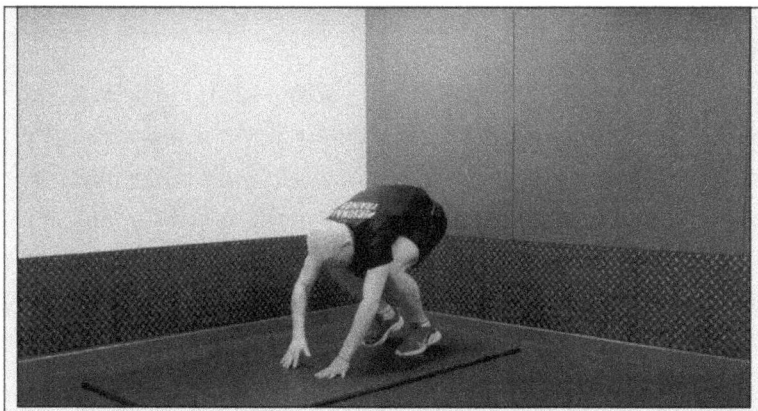

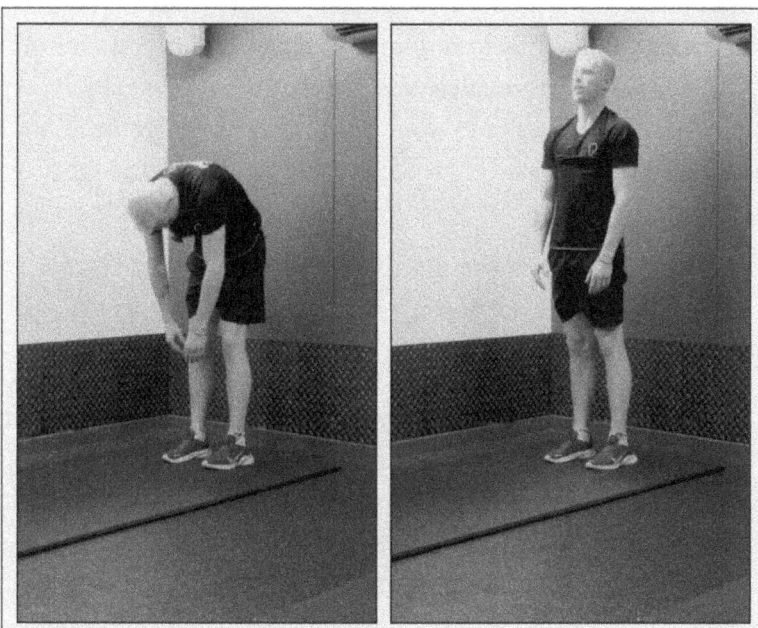

🔜 Return to the standing position.

Interactive Element: Create Your Dynamic Warm-Up Routine

Think about the activities you enjoy or the sports you play. Use the exercises mentioned to create your dynamic warm-up routine. Write down a sequence you can easily remember and perform before your workouts. Start with general movements like arm circles and leg swings. Then, move to more specific stretches, like walking lunges with a twist. Try it out and adjust as needed. Pay attention to how your body feels. This personalized routine will ensure you're ready for any physical activity.

Dynamic stretching is a powerful tool in your fitness arsenal. It's about more than just warming up. It prepares your body for movement, enhances performance, and reduces injury risks. By incorporating these stretches into your routine, you set yourself up for success. You'll be ready to tackle any workout or sport with confidence.

7.1 ACTIVATION EXERCISES FOR TARGETED MUSCLE GROUPS

Muscle activation is the key to waking up your muscles before they get to work. Think of it like starting a car engine on a cold morning. You want everything running smoothly before hitting the road. Activation exercises ensure that specific muscles are ready for more intense activity. When your muscles are correctly activated, they perform better. They can lift more, run faster, and endure longer. Glute bridges are a great way to activate your lower body. Lie on your back, bend your knees, and lift your hips. This exercise engages your glutes and prepares them for action. For your shoulders, try scapular push-ups. They help engage the muscles around your shoulder blades, making them stable and strong.

Let's talk about different exercises for various muscle groups. Clamshells are perfect for targeting your hip abductors. Lie on your side with your knees bent. Lift your top knee while keeping your feet together. This movement strengthens the muscles outside your hips, improving stability. For your upper back, band pull-aparts work wonders. Stand with your feet shoulder-width apart and hold a resistance band in front of you. Pull the band apart, keeping your arms straight. This exercise activates your upper back muscles, preparing them for lifting or pulling movements. These targeted activation routines ensure your muscles are ready to handle the demands of your workout.

Pre-activation exercises offer many benefits. They enhance muscle recruitment during your main exercises. This means your muscles work together more effectively, giving you more power and control. For example, activating your core before a workout helps you lift heavier weights safely. It reduces the risk of muscle strains and imbalances, which are common when muscles are not adequately engaged. When muscles are activated, they respond better to the demands of exercise. This reduces the chances of injury and improves overall performance. Pre-activation exercises are like giving your muscles a head start, setting the stage for a successful workout.

Consider incorporating sample activation routines into your workouts. For a lower body strength day, start with glute bridges and clamshells. These exercises wake up your glutes and hips, preparing them for squats and lunges. Follow with calf raises to activate your calves and improve balance. Begin with scapular push-ups and band pull-apart for upper-body and shoulder workouts. These exercises engage your shoulders and upper back, preparing them for pressing or pulling movements. Add some arm circles to warm up your arms and shoulders. These routines ensure your muscles are primed and ready, reducing the risk of injury.

Step 1: Starting Position (Glute Bridge)

Lie on your back with your knees bent, feet flat on the floor, hip-width apart.

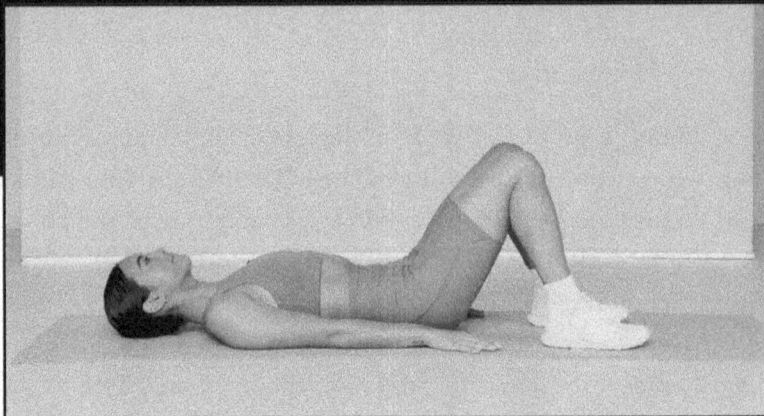

Keep your arms at your sides and engage your core to stabilize your lower back.

Step 2: Lifting the Hips

Push through your heels and lift your hips off the floor, aiming to form a straight line from your knees to your shoulders.

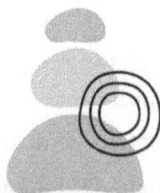

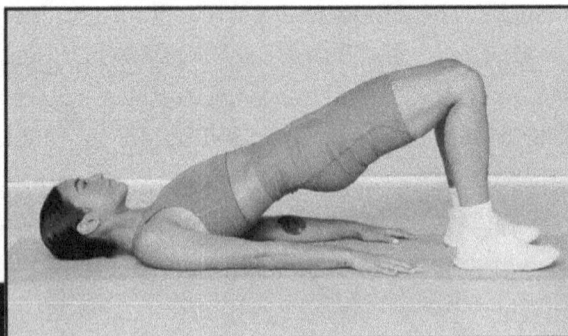

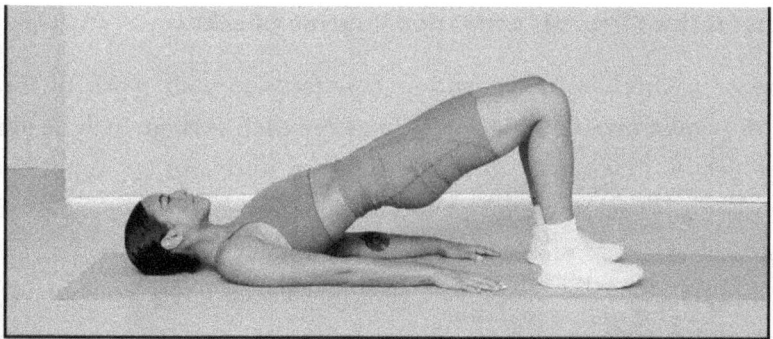

Step 3: Lower Your Hips

🔰 Slowly lower your hips back down to the floor, focusing on maintaining control.

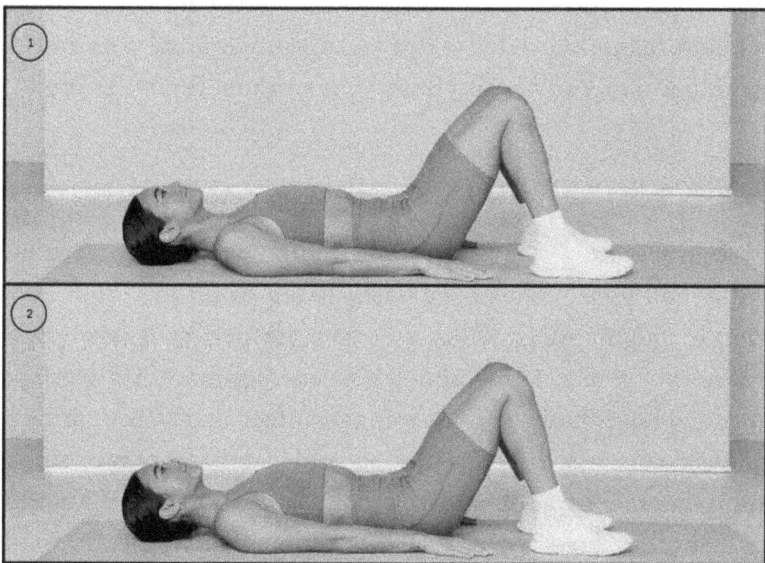

🔰 Perform 12 repetitions, holding at the top for 2-3 seconds each time. Perform 10-12 reps of both the inchworm and glute bridge.

Interactive Element: Activation Routine Checklist

Create a checklist of activation exercises for your workout days. Write down the exercises you'll do before each session. Include glute bridges for lower body days and scapular push-ups for upper body workouts. Check them off as you complete each one. This helps you remember the exercises and ensures you don't skip this critical step. A simple checklist keeps you accountable and sets you up for a successful workout.

Muscle activation is a small but crucial part of your fitness routine. It prepares your body for the challenges ahead, reducing injury risk and improving performance. Incorporate these exercises into your warm-up, and you'll notice a difference in how your body responds. It's about taking those few extra minutes to activate your muscles, ensuring you're ready for anything your workout throws at you.

7.2 INCORPORATING LOW-IMPACT CARDIO

Low-impact cardio exercises offer a gentle way to keep your heart healthy and your body strong without the strain that high-impact activities might bring. These exercises are perfect if you want to protect your joints. Think about how rowing machines work your upper and lower body while keeping your feet steady. Your arms pull and push, your legs drive the motion, and your heart pumps steadily. This makes rowing a full-body workout that's kind on the knees and hips. Another great option is the elliptical machine. It mimics walking or running but without the hard impact on your joints. Your feet stay on the pedals, and your body moves smoothly and continuously. This exercise is excellent for your cardiovascular health, helping you build endurance while being gentle on your body.

Some fun low-impact cardio exercises can give you the benefits of a good workout. Swimming is an excellent choice. The water supports your weight, so you can move freely without putting stress on your joints. Swimming laps strengthens your muscles and boosts your endurance. It's like giving your whole body a workout in one go. Cycling is another effective option. Whether on a stationary bike or exploring trails, cycling builds endurance and tones your legs. The movements are smooth, and the intensity can be adjusted to fit your level. Both swimming and cycling are activities you can enjoy alone or with friends. They provide variety and keep your exercise routine exciting.

Adding low-impact cardio to your weekly routine can balance your workout plan. It's important to schedule these sessions alongside other exercises. For example, you might cycle on days you're not lifting weights. This balances your exercise routine and gives your body time to recover from strength training. Combining low-impact cardio with strength workouts creates a well-rounded plan. You keep your heart fit while building muscle strength. It's a great way to improve your overall fitness without overloading any one part of your body. This approach helps you avoid burnout and keeps exercise enjoyable.

Consider a few strategies to get the most out of your low-impact cardio sessions. Interval training can add variety and intensity to your workouts. Instead of maintaining a steady pace, alternate between higher and lower intensity periods. For example, during a cycling session, you might pedal faster for one minute and then slow down for two minutes. This technique burns calories efficiently and boosts your endurance. Music can also enhance your workouts. Create a playlist with upbeat songs that motivate you. The rhythm can help you keep pace and make the session more enjoyable. A good playlist can turn a simple workout into an energizing experience.

Low-impact cardio exercises are versatile and can fit into any lifestyle. They offer a way to stay active while being gentle on your body. Whether you choose to row, swim, or cycle, you're taking steps to improve your health. These exercises help you stay fit, reduce stress, and enjoy a more active life. They remind you that exercise doesn't have to be hard on your body to be effective. You can achieve your fitness goals with enjoyable activities that are easy to stick with.

7.3 ADVANCED CORE STABILIZATION TECHNIQUES

Developing core strength goes beyond the basics. It involves exercises that challenge your stability and strength in new ways. One such exercise is the Pallof press. This move focuses on anti-rotational strength. Stand next to a cable machine, holding the handle with both hands at chest level. The cable pulls from one side, but your task is to keep your torso still while extending your arms straight out and pulling them back in. This exercise is simple yet effective. It strengthens your core by resisting rotation, which is crucial for maintaining balance and stability in everyday activities.

Another exercise that targets dynamic engagement is the standing cable woodchop. This move mimics chopping wood, engaging your core through a full range of motion. Stand with your feet shoulder-width apart, and hold the cable handle with both hands above one shoulder. Pull the cable diagonally across your body to your opposite hip. This movement works your core muscles while also engaging your shoulders and hips. It improves rotational strength and coordination, which is essential for sports and physical activities requiring twisting and turning.

Balance and coordination play a key role in core training. Single-leg deadlifts are an excellent way to enhance these skills. Stand on one leg, keeping the other slightly bent. Lean forward, reaching toward the ground with one hand while extending the opposite leg behind you. This exercise challenges your balance and strengthens your core, hamstrings, and glutes. It's perfect for improving stability and control. Bosu ball exercises add an extra layer of difficulty. When you perform exercises like squats or planks on a Bosu ball, your body must work harder to maintain balance. This engages your core and improves proprioception, which is your body's ability to sense its position and movement.

As you progress, you can increase the difficulty of core exercises. Start with bare planks, then move to plank variations. Try side planks or planks with arm raises to challenge your stability. Adding instability with equipment like Swiss balls can make exercises more challenging. When you do push-ups or sit-ups on a Swiss ball, your core engages more to keep you stable. This increases the effectiveness of your workouts and helps you build a stronger core. Progressing in this way ensures your muscles continue to develop, adapting to new challenges and building resilience.

Core stabilization routines can be tailored to specific goals. To enhance athletic performance, focus on exercises that improve power and agility. Incorporate explosive movements like medicine ball throws or jump squats. These exercises build strength and speed, which are essential for athletes. If your goal is injury prevention in daily activities, choose exercises emphasizing stability and control. Perform routines that include planks, bridges, and leg raises. These moves strengthen the core muscles that support your spine and protect against back pain. Focusing on specific objectives can make your core training more effective and relevant to your needs.

Visual Element: Core Workout Progression Chart

Create a visual chart to track your core workout progressions. Start with basic exercises like planks and single-leg deadlifts. As you gain strength, move to more challenging variations like side planks and Bosu ball exercises. Check off each progression as you master it. This chart provides a clear path for improvement and keeps you motivated as you advance in your core training.

Integrating these advanced techniques into your routine takes your core training to the next level. These exercises build strength and stability and enhance balance and coordination. Whether you aim to improve athletic performance or prevent injuries, these techniques provide the tools you need to succeed. With dedication and practice, you'll notice a stronger, more resilient core that supports all your activities.

7.4 COMBINING THERAPEUTIC EXERCISES WITH REGULAR WORKOUTS

Blending therapeutic exercises with your regular workout routine can transform your fitness experience. It's like having the best of both worlds in one session. Therapeutic exercises focus on healing and correcting imbalances. They strengthen weak areas and improve flexibility. Regular workouts focus on building strength, endurance, and cardiovascular fitness. By combining these approaches, you enhance your overall wellness. You target specific weaknesses while still building on your existing strengths. This combination addresses your body's needs, helping you become stronger and more balanced.

The structure is key to seamlessly integrating these different exercises. Consider alternating between therapeutic and high-intensity intervals. Start with a therapeutic exercise to activate and engage muscles. Follow it with a high-intensity burst to elevate your heart rate. This method keeps your body guessing and your mind engaged. Scheduling specific days for therapeutic focus is also beneficial. Dedicate certain days to exercises that focus on recovery and flexibility. Use the rest of the week for strength and cardio. This balance ensures that your body gets the attention it needs, reducing the risk of injury and promoting recovery. It allows you to enjoy a wide range of physical activities without overloading any one system.

Taking a holistic approach to fitness brings many benefits. By integrating different types of exercises, you improve cardiovascular health while supporting muscle recovery. For instance, pair a gentle yoga session with a brisk walk. The yoga promotes flexibility and relaxation, while walking boosts your heart health. This combination enhances physical and mental well-being. It provides a balanced routine that keeps you motivated. Varied activities prevent workout monotony and keep you excited about exercise. They also promote mental clarity and stress relief, essential for overall health.

Creating a balanced workout plan involves careful planning. Consider a weekly schedule that includes both therapeutic and regular exercises. For example, start the week with a focus on strength training. Follow this with a day dedicated to flexibility and core exercises. Midweek, include a cardio session to keep your heart strong. Later in the week, blend therapeutic exercises with light aerobic activity. This might consist of walking or swimming. Each session complements the others, creating a well-rounded routine. This plan supports all aspects of health, from strength and endurance to flexibility and recovery. It ensures your body gets the variety it needs to stay strong and resilient.

For your daily routines, think about how to mix these exercises seamlessly. Begin with a warm-up that includes both dynamic stretches and muscle activation. This prepares your body for more intense activity. As you move into your main workout, alternate between exercises. For instance, follow a set of lunges with a gentle stretch or core activation exercise. This keeps your muscles engaged without overworking them. After your workout, cool down with therapeutic movements that promote recovery and flexibility. This approach ensures you get the most out of each session, leaving you feeling balanced and energized.

The beauty of combining therapeutic and regular exercises lies in their synergy. Together, they create a comprehensive approach to health and fitness. They address the unique needs of your body while promoting overall wellness. This integration not only enhances physical performance but also contributes to mental well-being. By embracing this balanced approach, you create a fitness routine that supports a healthy, active lifestyle. It's about finding harmony in movement, where each exercise complements the next, building a stronger, healthier you. This chapter provided a roadmap for integrating therapeutic exercises into your routine. As you progress, explore new ways to challenge and support your body. These strategies will serve you well as you continue your journey toward lifelong fitness and well-being.

SEATED FORWARD FOLD (THERAPEUTIC STRETCH)

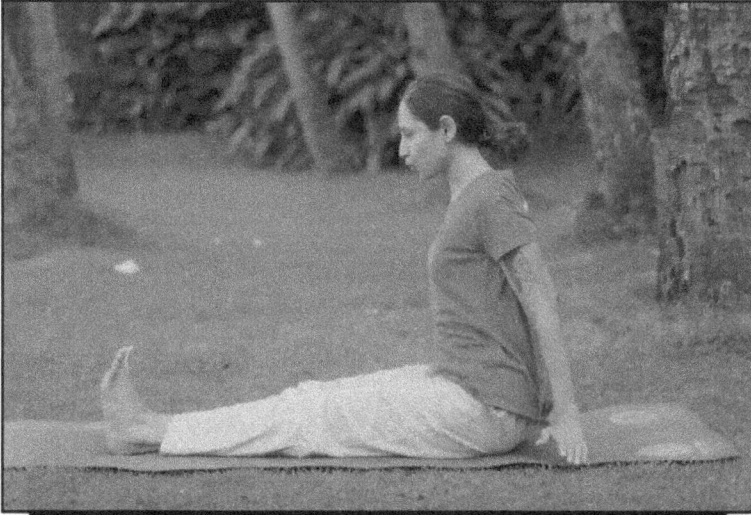

Step 1: Starting Position

➥ Sit on the floor with your legs extended straight in front of you and feet flexed.

➥ Keep your spine straight and arms by your sides.

Step 2: Reach Forward

➥ Inhale to lengthen your spine, then exhale as you hinge forward from your hips.

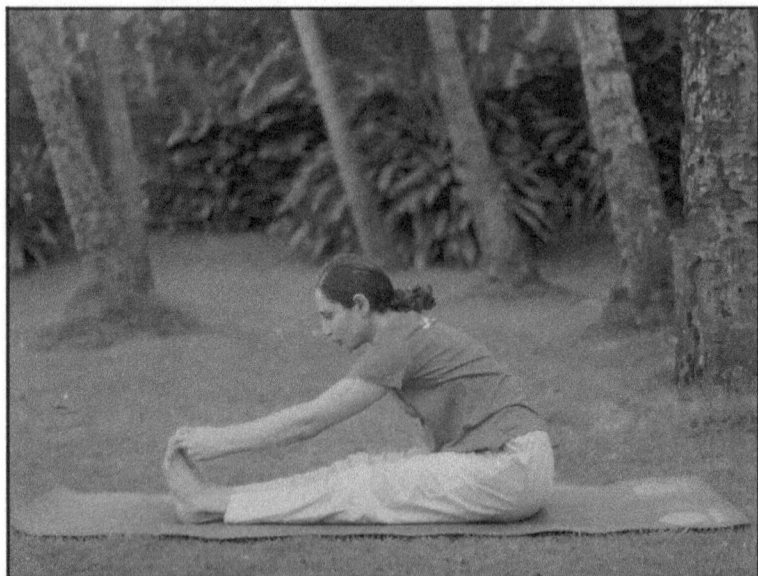

- Reach your hands toward your feet, shins, or ankles, depending on your flexibility.

- Allow your torso to gently rest over your legs, feeling a stretch in the hamstrings and lower back.

Step 3: Hold and Breathe

- Hold the stretch for 20-30 seconds, breathing deeply into the stretch.

- Focus on relaxing into the pose with each breath.

8

ADDRESSING COMMON CONCERNS AND QUESTIONS

———

I magine this: You've been sidelined by an injury, but now, you're eager to return to moving and feel like yourself again. It's a common scenario for many adults who are caught between wanting to stay active and fearing re-injury. Navigating this path requires a careful approach. Returning to exercise should be gradual, emphasizing safety and controlled progress. Jumping back into intense workouts too quickly can lead to setbacks. Instead, start with low-intensity exercises. These exercises allow your body to adjust without overwhelming it. Focus on controlled movements and proper form to rebuild strength and confidence. This cautious approach respects your body's healing process and creates a solid foundation for future activity.

Recognizing when you're ready to exercise again is crucial. You should notice the absence of sharp or persistent pain. Achieving baseline mobility and strength signals readiness, meaning you can move comfortably and perform basic tasks without discomfort. These indicators suggest that your body is prepared to handle more activity. It's essential to listen to what your body is telling you. If you're unsure, consult with a healthcare provider. They can offer guidance and help you determine your readiness for exercise. They might recommend specific exercises that align with your recovery stage, ensuring you don't push too hard too soon.

Monitoring your body's response to exercise is key to a triumphant return. Keeping an exercise log is a simple yet effective tool. Note how you feel during and after workouts, paying attention to any pain levels. This log acts as a diary, helping you track progress and identify recurring issues. Regularly consult with healthcare providers to review your log. They can provide valuable insights and adjust your routine as needed. This ongoing communication ensures that your recovery stays on track and you promptly address any concerns. By being proactive, you minimize the risk of setbacks and build confidence in your recovery journey.

8.1 CHECKLIST FOR SAFE EXERCISE PRACTICES

1. **Warm-up and Cool-down Routines:** Begin each session with a gentle warm-up to prepare your muscles. End with a cool-down to ease your body back to rest.
2. **Proper Hydration and Nutrition:** Drink water before, during, and after exercise. Fuel your body with nutritious foods that support healing and energy.
3. **Controlled Movements:** Focus on slow, deliberate actions. Avoid sudden or jerky movements that can strain healing tissues.
4. **Consistent Rest:** Allow your body time to recover between sessions. Rest days are essential for healing and strength-building.
5. **Listen to Your Body:** If something feels wrong, stop. Pain is a signal to pause and reassess your approach.

By following these guidelines, you create a safe environment for exercise. This checklist serves as a reminder to prioritize your health and well-being as you ease back into physical activity.

Returning to exercise after an injury involves patience and attentiveness. It's about rebuilding your strength and confidence without rushing. Embrace this process as an opportunity to learn more about your body and its capabilities. Stay mindful of your progress and celebrate each milestone, no matter how small. This careful approach not only aids recovery but also sets the stage for sustained health and vitality in the long run.

8.2 MODIFYING EXERCISES FOR LIMITED MOBILITY

Imagine a world where moving easily is within everyone's reach, regardless of mobility. Traditional exercises can seem daunting for many adults, especially with limited movement. However, adapting exercises makes fitness accessible to all. One effective strategy is to use chairs or supports for stability. This approach allows you to perform exercises without straining or risking injury. For instance, using a chair to support your body during squats can help you maintain balance while engaging your leg muscles. It provides confidence and safety, especially when starting. Performing movements while seated or lying down opens up a world of possibilities. Seated exercises can be just as practical as standing ones. You can do simple leg lifts or seated marches to keep your body active. Lying down exercises, like leg raises or gentle core work, also offer a comfortable way to engage muscles without added pressure on your joints.

The right equipment can significantly enhance your exercise routine. Resistance bands are fantastic tools for gentle stretching. They allow you to add resistance to your movements without needing heavy weights. You can sit and perform simple arm or leg stretches with a band. This helps improve strength and flexibility. Foam rollers are another great tool for support and balance. They are excellent for releasing tension in tight muscles and improving circulation. You can use them to massage sore areas gently or to assist in balance exercises. These tools provide support and versatility, making them ideal for anyone modifying their workout routine.

Modified exercises offer numerous health benefits. They can improve circulation by getting their blood flowing, which is vital for overall health. When you move, your heart pumps blood more efficiently, delivering oxygen and nutrients to your cells. This boost in circulation helps your body function better. Flexibility also increases as you incorporate these exercises into your routine. Regular movement keeps your joints mobile and muscles supple. This reduces stiffness and makes daily tasks easier. Beyond physical benefits, exercise can enhance mental well-being. Engaging in physical activity releases endorphins, the body's natural mood boosters. These chemicals help reduce stress and improve your mood, leaving you feeling more positive and energized.

There are many ways to adapt common exercises to fit your needs. Chair yoga is a perfect example. It adapts traditional yoga poses to a seated position, focusing on flexibility and balance. You can perform poses like seated forward folds or gentle twists right from your chair. These movements stretch your muscles and calm your mind, making them great for relaxation. Seated strength training with light weights is another option. You can do bicep curls or shoulder presses while sitting. This builds upper body strength without straining your legs. Using light weights reduces the risk of injury while still challenging your muscles. These adaptations ensure you stay active and engaged without compromising your safety.

Exercise doesn't have to be complicated or demanding. It's about finding what works for you and making it part of your routine. With the proper modifications, you can enjoy the benefits of physical activity regardless of mobility challenges. Whether you use supports or try seated exercises, the key is to keep moving. Movement is a powerful tool for improving health and boosting mood. Embracing these adaptations opens the door to a healthier, more active lifestyle.

SEATED MARCHES WITH RESISTANCE BANDS

Step 1: Starting Position

⌁ Sit on a chair with your feet flat on the floor and the resistance band placed around your thighs.

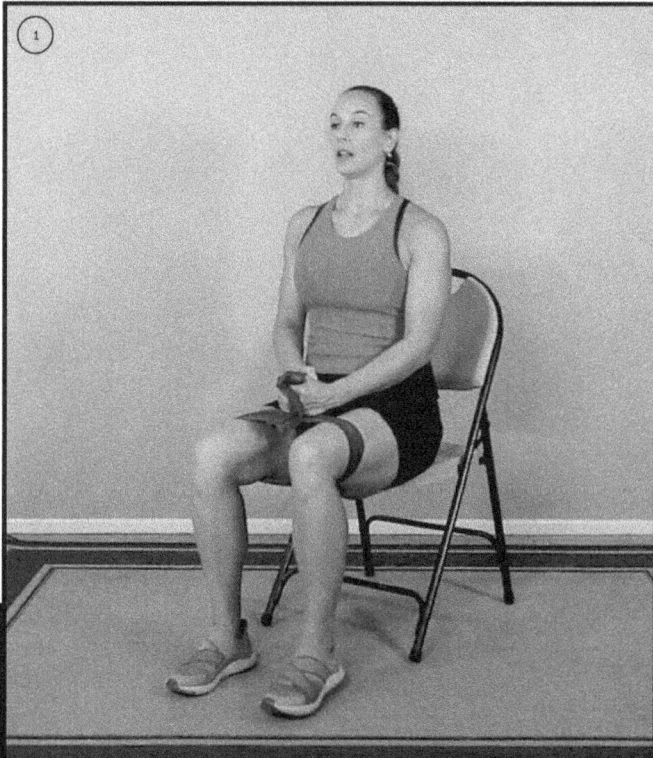

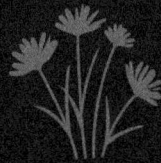

Step 2: Marching with Band

⟳ Lift your right knee toward your chest while resisting the pull of the band.

⟳ Alternate legs while maintaining good posture.

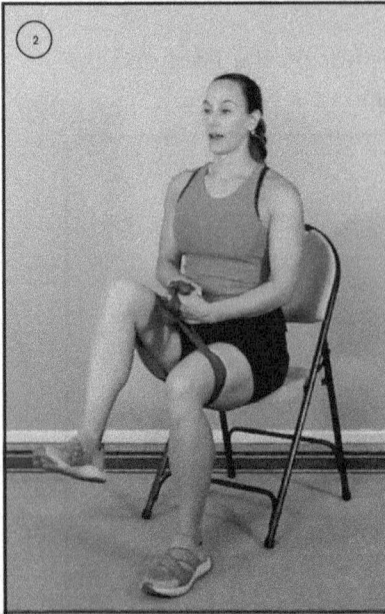

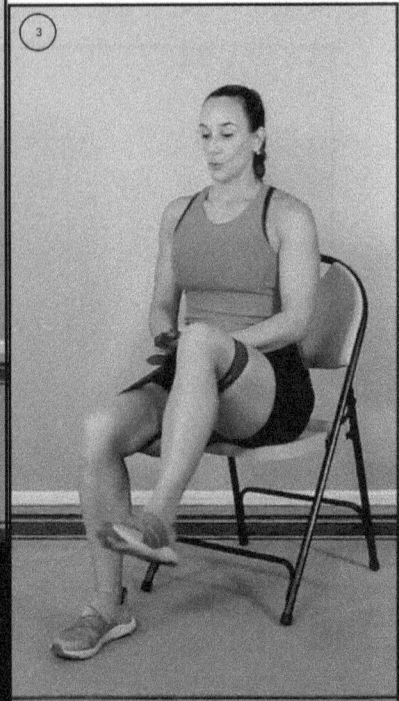

Step 3: Intensity Adjustment:

➤ Increase or decrease the resistance by adjusting the tension of the band.

➤ Perform 30 seconds per leg, focusing on controlled movements.

8.3 PAIN MANAGEMENT DURING EXERCISE

When you exercise, it's normal to feel some discomfort. This is often a sign that your muscles are adapting and getting stronger. We call this muscle soreness. It usually shows up a day or two after a workout and is a part of the process. However, it's crucial to distinguish this from pain that signals harm. Sharp pain, on the other hand, is a red flag. It can mean something is wrong. If you feel a sudden, intense pain that doesn't disappear, you must stop what you're doing. This type of pain can indicate an injury that needs attention.

Managing pain during exercise is about knowing what to do when discomfort arises. One effective technique is applying heat or ice after your workout. Heat can relax tight muscles and improve blood flow. This is helpful when you're feeling stiff. Ice, on the other hand, can reduce swelling and acute pain. It's beneficial if you've pushed too hard and your joints are sore. Incorporating rest days into your routine is another key strategy. Giving your body time to recover is essential for avoiding injuries. Active recovery days, where you engage in light activities like walking or gentle stretching, can also keep your body moving without the strain of a complete workout.

Mind-body techniques play a significant role in managing pain. Practices like mindfulness help you stay aware of your body's signals. Breathing exercises are a simple way to bring relaxation and focus during discomfort. Deep, slow breaths can calm your nervous system and reduce the sensation of pain. Visualization techniques are also powerful. Picture yourself completing your exercises with ease, focusing on each movement. This mental imagery can enhance your ability to cope with discomfort, making your workout experience more positive and effective. These techniques help with pain and improve your overall mental well-being.

There are times when seeking professional help becomes necessary. Persistent or worsening symptoms are signs that shouldn't be ignored. If pain affects your daily activities or you notice it increasing over time, it's time to consult a healthcare professional. They can assess your situation and recommend appropriate treatment. This might include physical therapy, adjustments to your exercise routine, or even rest. Remember, it's always better to err on the side of caution. Addressing pain early can prevent more serious issues and ensure you stay on the path to health and fitness.

8.4 INCORPORATING EXERCISE INTO BUSY SCHEDULES

Life can feel like a constant race against the clock. With work, family, and endless to-dos, finding time to exercise often falls to the bottom of the list. But staying active doesn't have to mean setting aside hours each day. Instead, prioritize short, high-intensity workouts that fit into your schedule. These workouts, often called HIIT (high-intensity interval training), pack a big punch in a short amount of time. They get your heart pumping and muscles working in 20 to 30 minutes. Consider waking up just a little earlier if you have a busy morning. A quick session before your day starts can leave you feeling energized and ready for what's ahead.

Another strategy is to utilize breaks throughout your day. Quick exercise sessions during lunch or between meetings can make a big difference. You don't need a gym or special equipment. Use your body weight for push-ups, squats, or jumping jacks. These moves can be done anywhere and don't require much space. Even a five-minute stretching routine can refresh your body and mind. These short bursts of activity keep you moving and help manage stress. They remind you that staying active is possible, no matter how packed your schedule is.

The concept of micro-workouts can change how you think about exercise. Instead of one long session, break it into smaller parts. Five-minute routines can add up throughout the day. Try a quick body-weight circuit in the morning, a brisk walk during lunch, and some stretching before bed. These small efforts add up to significant benefits. They keep your metabolism active and your energy levels up. Micro-workouts also fit into your lifestyle without overwhelming it. They show that every bit of movement counts, proving you don't need a lot of time to make a significant impact on your health.

Creating a schedule that works for you is key. Morning workouts might be your best bet if you're an early riser. Start your day with a quick run or a series of yoga poses. This boosts your mood and sets a positive tone for the day. For those who prefer midday activity, a lunchtime session can break up your workday and clear your mind. Whether it's a walk outside or a short gym visit, this time recharges your batteries. Evening workouts offer flexibility, too. They help unwind and relieve stress after a long day. Choose whatever time fits best into your routine, and most importantly, keep it consistent.

To make it easier, consider planning your week. Look at your schedule and find pockets of time to fit in exercise. Monday and Wednesday mornings may be best for cardio, while Tuesday and Thursday evenings work for strength training. Keep your plan visible on a calendar or a note on your phone. This visual reminder keeps you accountable and motivated. Remember, the best workout is the one you can stick to. Adapt your plan as needed, and don't be too hard on yourself if life gets in the way. Flexibility is key to maintaining an active lifestyle.

Step 1: Neck Tilts

Slowly tilt your head to each side, holding for a few second.

Perform 5-6 reps per side.

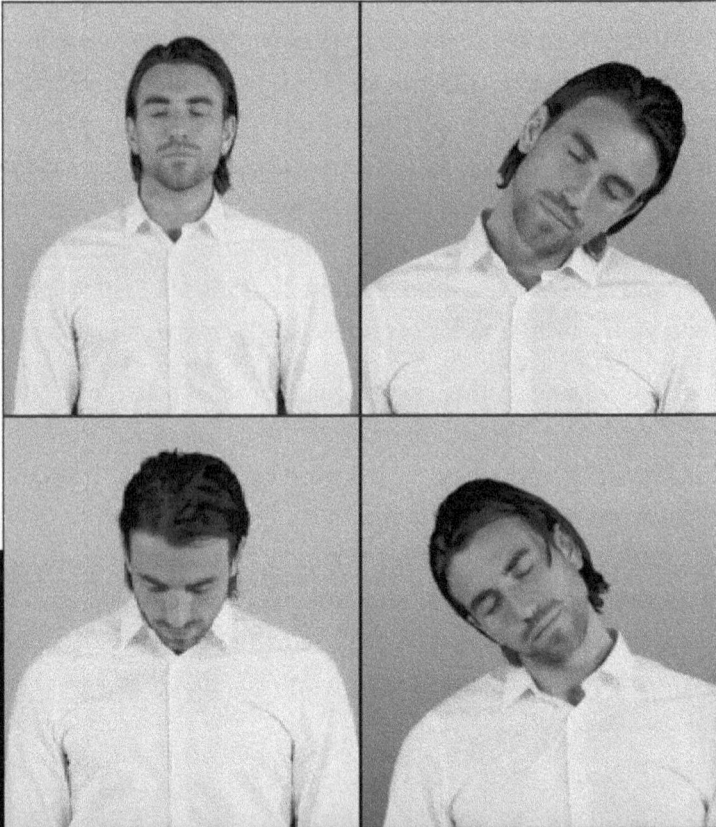

Step 1: Shoulder Shrugs

⁖ Raise shoulders to ears, hold, and lower.

⁖ Perform 8-10 reps.

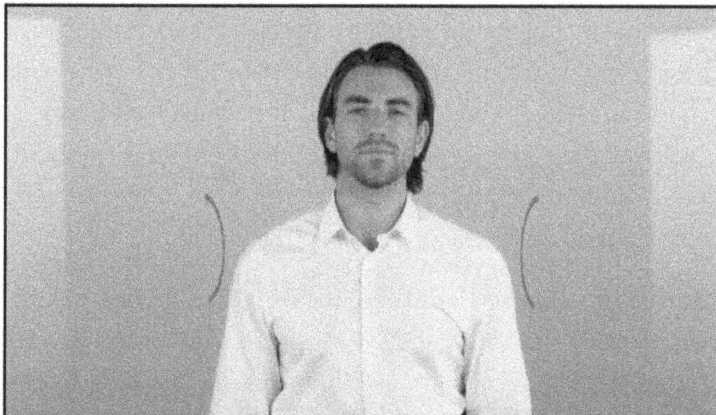

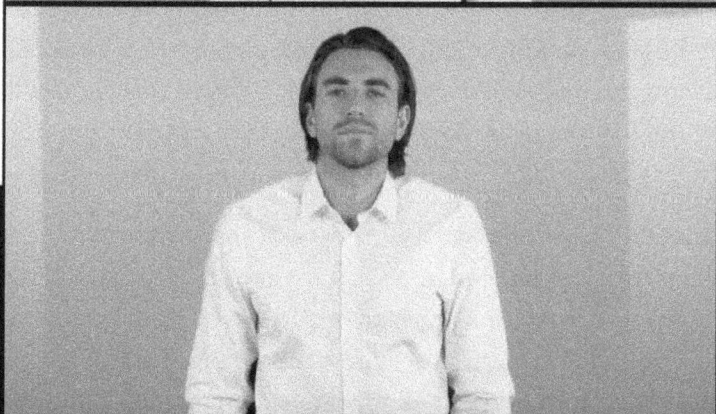

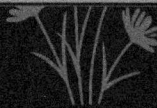

8.5 EVALUATING ONLINE RESOURCES FOR CREDIBILITY

In today's world, the internet is full of fitness tips and exercise advice. But not all of it is helpful or safe. It's essential to know how to find reliable information. Start by checking the author's credentials and expertise. A qualified author usually has a background in health or fitness. They might hold degrees or certifications in related fields. This shows they know what they're talking about. Also, check if their work is backed by peer-reviewed and published studies. Experts in the field review these studies. This ensures the information is accurate and trustworthy.

Misinformation can be harmful. Following bad advice can lead to injury. For example, using the wrong form during an exercise can cause strains or sprains. Some online articles exaggerate exercise benefits. They promise quick fixes or miraculous results. This can create false expectations and disappointment. Always be cautious if something sounds too good to be true. It often is. Misleading claims can waste your time and money. Worse, they can hurt your health. It's vital to stay informed and skeptical.

Fortunately, there are tools to help you verify information. Fact-checking websites are a great resource. They often review claims and provide evidence for or against them. These sites help separate fact from fiction. Another strategy is to consult with healthcare professionals. They have the training and experience to offer reliable advice. Ask a doctor or physical therapist if you're unsure about something you've read online. They can confirm whether the advice is safe and effective. This extra step can save you from potential harm.

Critical thinking is your best defense against misinformation. Always question the motivations behind online publications. Ask yourself why the information is being shared. Is the author trying to sell a product or service? This could bias their advice. Also, seek multiple perspectives. Look for different articles or studies on the same topic. This gives you a balanced view and helps you make informed decisions. Developing a skeptical mindset ensures you only follow credible advice.

As this chapter ends, remember that informed decisions lead to better outcomes. The following section will explore deepening your knowledge and expanding your skills through advanced techniques.

9

HOLISTIC APPROACHES TO THERAPEUTIC EXERCISE

P icture this: you've just finished a challenging workout. You feel the sweat on your skin and the burn in your muscles. But there's something else that can help you feel even better. It's not a fancy gadget or a new exercise technique. It's the food you eat. Nutrition plays a massive role in how your body recovers. It's like the fuel that powers your body's repair shop. After you exercise, your muscles need help to heal and grow stronger. This is where nutrition steps in.

When you exercise, your muscles undergo tiny tears. This might sound alarming, but it's a natural part of building strength. Your body repairs these tears, making your muscles stronger than before. Protein is a key player in this process. It provides the building blocks your muscles need to repair and grow. Foods rich in protein, like chicken, fish, and legumes, are excellent choices. They help rebuild muscle tissue and support overall recovery. But protein isn't the only nutrient that matters. Carbohydrates play a vital role, too. They replenish your energy stores, allowing you to recover faster and feel more energized for your next workout.

Hydration is another crucial aspect of recovery. When you exercise, you lose fluids through sweat. Replacing these fluids is essential. Water helps transport nutrients to your cells. It also aids in digestion and regulates body temperature. Staying hydrated supports your body's recovery processes. It ensures that every system functions smoothly. Make sure to drink water before, during, and after exercise. This simple habit can make a big difference in how you feel and recover.

Incorporating nutrient-rich foods into your diet can further enhance recovery. Lean proteins, like those mentioned earlier, are a great start. But don't forget about fruits and vegetables. They are packed with antioxidants. Antioxidants help combat inflammation and speed up recovery. Berries, oranges, and leafy greens are especially beneficial. They support your body's repair processes and boost your immune system. Eating various colorful fruits and vegetables ensures you get a wide range of nutrients. This keeps your body strong and healthy.

The timing of nutrient intake is also essential. Eating the right foods at the right time can maximize their benefits. Before a workout, have a meal or snack with protein and carbohydrates. This combination fuels your body and prepares it for exercise. After working out, focus on replenishing your energy stores. Eat a meal rich in protein and carbohydrates within an hour of finishing exercise. This helps repair muscles and restore glycogen levels. It also reduces muscle soreness, allowing you to bounce back quickly. By paying attention to when you eat, you can enhance your body's recovery and performance.

Nutritional deficiencies can hinder recovery and overall health. Iron and calcium are two nutrients that are often lacking. Iron is vital for carrying oxygen to your muscles. Without enough iron, you might feel tired and weak. Foods like red meat, beans, and spinach are good sources of iron. Calcium is essential for bone health. It helps maintain strong bones and prevents fractures. Dairy products, almonds, and broccoli are rich in calcium. Omega-3 fatty acids are another nutrient to consider. They reduce inflammation and support heart health. You'll find them in fish like salmon and in flaxseeds. Including these nutrients in your diet can improve recovery and keep your body functioning optimally.

Interactive Element: Nutritional Reflection Journal

Consider keeping a journal to track your nutrition and recovery. Write down what you eat and how you feel after workouts. Note any changes in energy levels or soreness. This reflection can help you identify patterns and make informed choices about your diet. It's a simple tool that provides valuable insights into how nutrition affects your recovery.

Understanding the connection between nutrition and recovery empowers you to make choices that support your health and fitness goals. You can optimize your recovery and performance by fueling your body with the proper nutrients at the correct times. Remember, what you put into your body is as important as how you move it.

Step 1: Starting Position

🦅 Start on your hands and knees, with your big toes touching and knees spread apart.

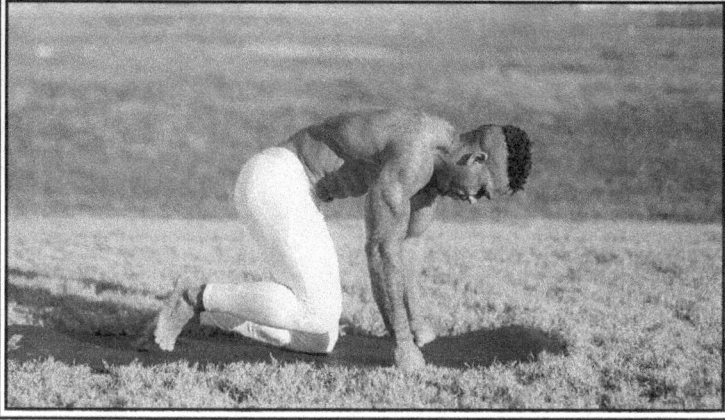

🦅 Slowly sit back onto your heels, bringing your chest toward the floor.

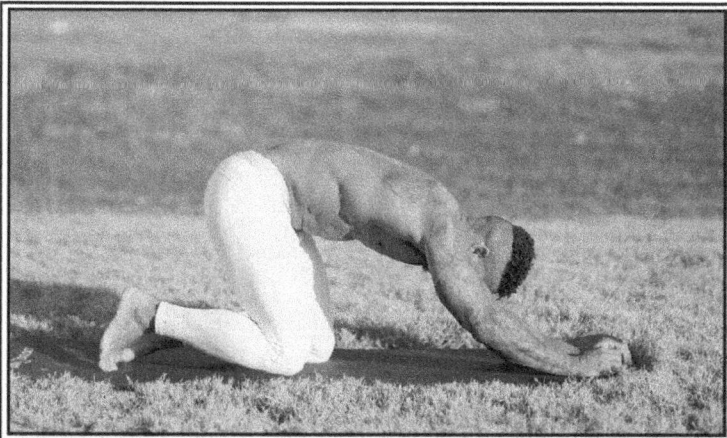

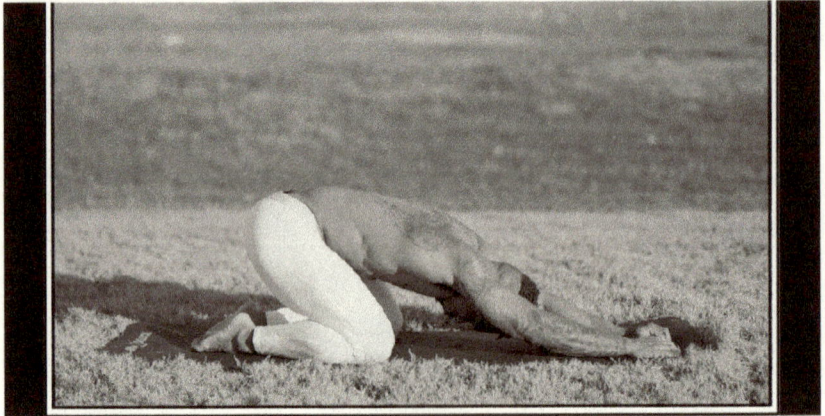

➥ Extend your arms forward on the mat.

➥ Breathe deeply, expanding your belly on the inhale and relaxing on the exhale.

➥ Hold for 15 seconds to 30 Seconds, then return to starting position.

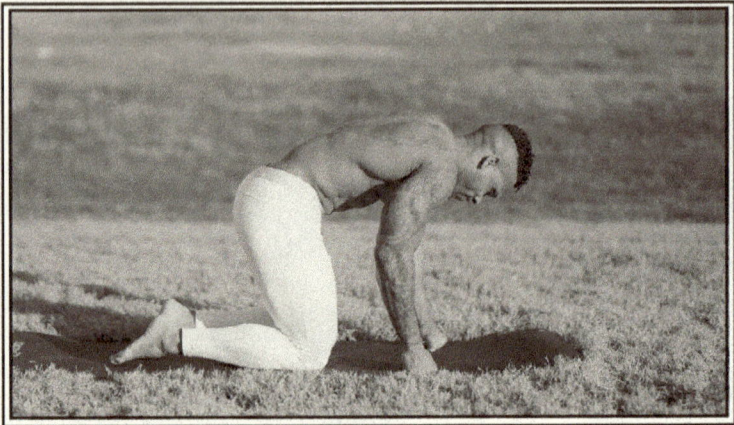

9.1 THE IMPORTANCE OF SLEEP AND REST

Imagine your body as a construction site. Every time you work out, you're like a builder tearing down old walls to make space for something more substantial. But to build effectively, you need quality materials and time to work. In this analogy, sleep is when your body's construction team gets to work. It is when your muscles repair and your body resets. During profound sleep, your body releases growth hormones. These hormones are like the supervisors on the site, directing repairs and rebuilding muscles. This process is vital for muscle repair and overall health. Without enough sleep, the construction work slows down, affecting your muscles and well-being.

Sleep also plays a critical role in maintaining hormonal balance. Hormones are like messengers that tell your body how to function. When you don't sleep well, these messengers get confused, leading to mood swings and increased stress. Over time, this imbalance can affect your physical health, too. It may lead to weight gain or a weakened immune system. Deep sleep is vital. It allows your body to manage stress and repair tissues. It's the stage where your body does most of its healing work, ensuring you wake up refreshed and ready for the day.

Improving your sleep quality is not just about getting more hours in bed. It's about ensuring those hours are restful. Establishing a consistent schedule is one of the best ways to improve sleep. Try going to bed and waking up at the same time every day. This routine helps regulate your body's internal clock, making it easier to fall asleep and wake up. Creating a restful environment is also key. Make your bedroom a peaceful space. Keep it calm, dark, and quiet. Remove distractions like bright lights or noisy electronics. These simple changes can help you drift into a deeper, more restorative sleep.

Rest is not just about sleep. It's also about giving your body a break from exercise. Rest days are crucial for recovery and progress. They give your muscles time to repair and grow. But the rest of the days don't mean you have to be completely inactive. Active recovery techniques can be very beneficial. Consider gentle activities like walking or stretching. These activities keep your blood flowing without putting stress on your muscles. They help reduce soreness and improve flexibility. Active recovery supports both physical and mental rejuvenation. It allows you to relax while still staying engaged in your fitness routine.

Ignoring the need for rest can lead to overtraining. This is when you push your body too hard without giving it enough time to recover. Overtraining can cause symptoms like fatigue, decreased performance, and even injuries. You might feel more tired than usual or notice that your workouts are getting more complex instead of easier. Your body may also become more susceptible to illnesses. Without rest, your immune system struggles to keep up, increasing the risk of colds or other infections. Listen to your body. If you notice these signs, it might be time to step back and rest.

Sleep deprivation is another risk associated with a lack of rest. It can affect your mood and cognitive functions. You might find it harder to concentrate or feel more irritable. Sleep deprivation can also impact your physical performance. Tasks that once seemed easy may feel more challenging. Your reaction times might slow, increasing the risk of accidents or injuries. To avoid these issues, prioritize rest and sleep as integral parts of your fitness plan. They are not just breaks from activity but essential components of a healthy lifestyle.

Recognizing the importance of sleep and rest in physical recovery is vital. They allow your body to repair, grow, and prepare for future challenges. By valuing rest, you support your overall health and enhance your performance. Make sleep a priority, and embrace rest days as part of your fitness routine. These practices will help you achieve your health goals more effectively and enjoy the process.

9.2 BALANCING PHYSICAL AND MENTAL HEALTH

Have you ever noticed how much better you feel after a good work-out? It's not just your imagination. Exercise releases chemicals in your brain called endorphins. These are often known as "feel-good" hormones. They help improve your mood and make you feel happier. When you move your body and get your heart pumping, these endorphins flood your brain, washing away stress and anxiety. This is one reason people often feel more positive and relaxed after exercising. Physical activity doesn't just boost your physical health. It also lifts your spirits and calms your mind.

Regular exercise can also lower anxiety and stress levels. When you're active, your body produces less stress hormone cortisol. High levels of cortisol can make you feel anxious or tense. By keeping this hormone in check, exercise helps you feel more at ease. Plus, focusing on your movements during a workout gives your mind a break from daily worries. It's like hitting the reset button, allowing you to approach problems with a clearer mind. This mental clarity can help you handle life's challenges more confidently and calmly.

Maintaining a balance between physical and mental well-being involves more than exercise. It's about taking care of your mental health, too. Scheduling regular mental health check-ins can help you stay in tune with yourself. Take a few moments each week to reflect on how you're feeling. Are there areas of your life causing stress? Are you feeling overwhelmed? These check-ins can help you identify issues early and find ways to address them. Incorporating mindfulness practices into your daily life also supports mental health. Simple techniques like deep breathing or meditation can help you stay grounded. They teach you to focus on the present moment, reducing stress and enhancing your overall well-being.

A strong mental state plays a crucial role in reaching your fitness goals. Visualization techniques can help you see yourself achieving your goals. Picture yourself completing that run or lifting those weights. This mental rehearsal boosts your confidence and motivation. Positive affirmations are another tool. These are short, positive statements you repeat to yourself. They can shift your mindset and keep you focused on your goals. For example, saying "I am strong and capable" can reinforce your belief in your abilities. These techniques help build mental resilience, pushing you through challenges and setbacks.

Finding support for your mental health is essential. If you're feeling stuck or overwhelmed, contact a mental health professional. They can provide guidance and support tailored to your needs. Therapy can offer valuable insights and coping strategies. It's a safe space to explore your thoughts and feelings. Joining support groups or online communities can also be beneficial. Connecting with others who share similar experiences can offer encouragement and understanding. These groups can become a source of motivation and inspiration. They remind you that you're not alone on your path to better health.

Textual Element: Resource List for Mental Health Support

Here are some resources to help you find mental health support. You might find helpful websites for locating therapists or online forums where you can connect with others. Check out local mental health organizations for support groups in your area. These resources can guide you in finding the help and community you need.

Taking care of your mental health is as important as your physical health. Exercise is a powerful tool that can improve both. By understanding the connection between your body and mind, you can create a balanced approach to wellness. Embrace practices that support your mental well-being. They will help you lead a happier and healthier life.

9.3 YOGA AND MEDITATION FOR ENHANCED WELL-BEING

Yoga can do a lot for both your body and mind. It can be a great addition to therapeutic exercise. When you practice yoga, you work on your flexibility and balance. These are important for everyday activities. Simple poses help stretch tight muscles and improve your range of motion. This can make moving around easier and help prevent injuries. Yoga is also about balance. Standing on one leg or moving slowly from one pose to another makes you more stable. This allows you to walk or do any physical activity.

But yoga isn't just about moving your body. It helps you relax, too. When you do yoga, you learn to control your breath. Deep breathing calms your mind and lowers stress. It's like taking a moment to pause and reset. This is important because stress can affect your health in many ways. Being able to manage it can help you feel better overall. By focusing on your breath, you also improve your concentration. This focus carries over into your daily life, making it easier to handle stress and stay calm.

Meditation is another part of yoga that helps with relaxation. In meditation, you sit quietly and focus on your breath or a word. This practice enables you to clear your mind. It teaches you to focus on the present moment instead of worrying about the past or future. This can help reduce stress and anxiety. It's like giving your brain a break from all the noise. Meditation can also help you focus better during workouts. When you're more focused, you can perform exercises with better form. This makes your workouts more effective and enjoyable.

Many yoga poses can support therapeutic exercise. One of them is the downward dog. This pose stretches your hamstrings and calves. It's excellent for improving flexibility in your legs. To do it, press your hands and feet into the ground, forming an upside-down V with your body. Another helpful pose is the child's pose. It's a gentle way to stretch your back and relax your mind. Kneel on the floor and sit back on your heels. Stretch your arms forward and rest your forehead on the ground. Both poses help you unwind and support your body's healing process.

Starting a yoga and meditation practice is easy, and you don't need much. First, think about what type of yoga you want to try. There are many styles, like gentle yoga or something more active. A beginner class is a good start if you're new to yoga. These classes focus on simple poses and teach you the basics. You can find classes at local studios or online. Online courses are convenient because you can do them at home. If you choose to start at home, create a space where you feel comfortable. You don't need a lot of room. Just enough to move freely. Place a yoga mat on the floor to keep you steady during poses. Keep the space quiet and free from distractions. This helps you focus during your practice.

You'll notice changes in your body and mind as you practice yoga and meditation. You might find that you're more flexible and balanced. Daily movements become more effortless. You may also feel calmer and more focused. These small changes add up, improving your overall well-being. Yoga and meditation are simple practices that can have a significant impact. They support both your physical health and mental clarity. Adding them to your routine gives you the tools to lead a healthier, more balanced life.

Step 1: Starting Position

🕊 Sit comfortably with your legs crossed, back straight, and hands resting on your knees.

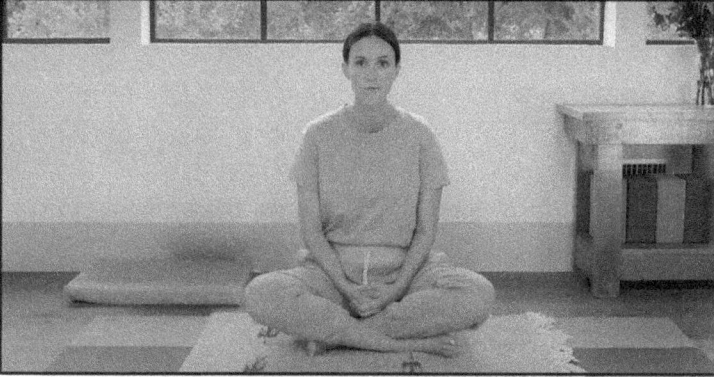

Step 2: Gentle Stretching

🕊 Begin with gentle stretches, such as a forward fold or seated side stretches, to release tension.

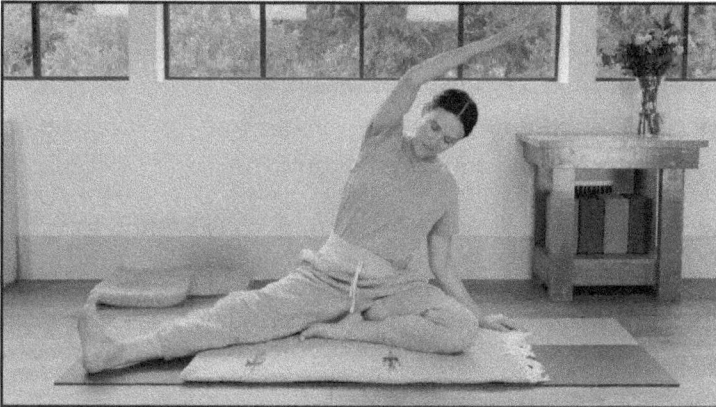

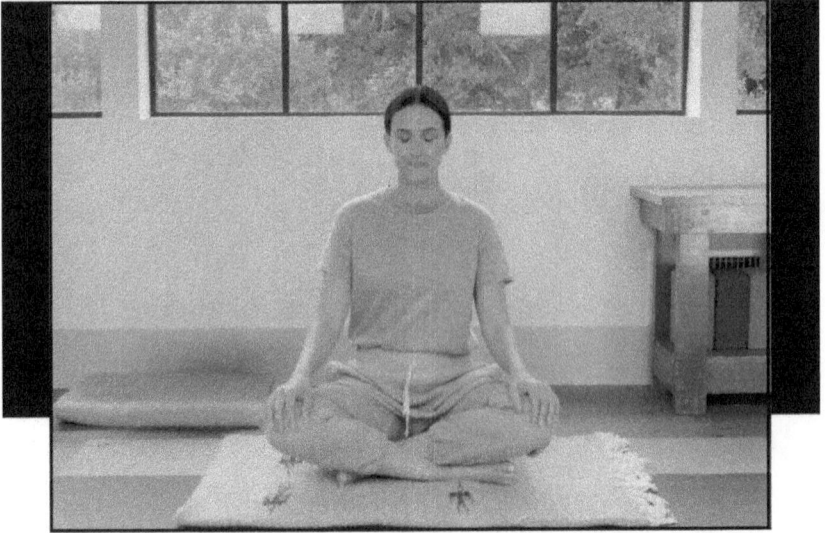

Step 3: Deep Breathing

🪷 Close your eyes, inhale deeply through your nose, and exhale through your mouth.

🪷 Focus on deep, rhythmic breathing for 5 minutes to calm your mind.

Step 4: Meditation

🪷 As you breathe deeply, focus on a positive affirmation or a calming thought.

🪷 Allow your body and mind to relax fully, letting go of any stress.

10

SUSTAINED SUCCESS AND LIFELONG WELLNESS

———

I magine you've found a rhythm in your life, a routine that flows effortlessly and supports your health. This isn't about grand gestures or extreme changes. It's about finding a balance that works for you and fits into your daily life. Creating a sustainable exercise routine is the key to lasting health and wellness. Let's explore how to develop a plan that keeps you moving forward without feeling overwhelmed. The goal is to craft a routine you can maintain over a lifetime, embracing changes and challenges.

Creating a realistic, long-term exercise plan means considering both intensity and duration. You want workouts that challenge you without leading to burnout. Finding the right balance is crucial. It's like cooking a meal; too much spice can ruin the dish, but just the right amount makes it delicious. Start with exercises that fit your fitness level and gradually increase their intensity. Focus on how your body feels. Listen to it and adjust as needed. Remember, it's not about how hard you push but how consistently you show up.

Periodizing your workouts is another way to keep things fresh and aligned with life's changes. This means varying your exercises according to the seasons or your life's demands. You may enjoy running outside in the summer, but prefer indoor activities like yoga in the winter. This flexibility helps you stay engaged and prevents boredom. Life is unpredictable, and your routine should be adaptable. Adjust your plan if your work schedule changes or you deal with family responsibilities. Fit in shorter workouts or modify them to suit your new circumstances. Adaptability is your ally in maintaining a lifelong fitness commitment.

Consider the idea of habit stacking. This technique helps you build new habits by linking them to existing ones. For example, add a quick set of squats while you brush your teeth. Or do stretches during TV commercials. This strategy uses your current habits as anchors for new ones. It makes changes feel less daunting and more natural. Habit stacking is about making small, manageable changes that add up over time. You can use reminders and cues, like setting alarms, to reinforce these habits until they become second nature.

Consistency matters more than perfection. It's about making regular activity a part of your life, even when things get hectic. Aim for small, consistent efforts rather than intense, irregular workouts. If you miss a session, don't sweat it. Focus on getting back to your routine as soon as you can. Celebrate the days you show up, even if it's just for a brief walk or a few stretches. This mindset shift encourages a positive relationship with fitness, emphasizing progress over perfection.

Interactive Element: Habit Stacking Exercise

Create a list of your daily habits, like drinking coffee or commuting. Identify opportunities to pair these with simple exercises. Write down a plan and place it where you'll see it often, such as on the fridge or near your workspace. Track your progress weekly to see how these small changes contribute to your overall wellness. This exercise helps you incorporate fitness into your life and shows how achievable and rewarding minor adjustments can be.

As you build your routine, remember that the journey to wellness is ongoing. Embrace the changes and growth that come with it. Your routine should evolve with you, supporting your goals and well-being. By focusing on sustainability, adaptability, and consistency, you create a foundation for lifelong health and vitality.

10.1 EMBRACING A LIFESTYLE OF MOVEMENT

Imagine a world where every step you take counts towards better health. Movement doesn't have to mean hitting the gym; it can be part of your everyday life. When you think about it, there are many opportunities to move more. Walking or cycling instead of driving is a simple change that can make a big difference. Not only does it improve your fitness, but it helps the environment, too. You get fresh air, save money on gas, and enjoy the world around you. These small changes create a more active lifestyle without much effort.

Choosing active leisure activities can also transform how you spend your free time. Why not try something different instead of sitting in front of the TV? Hiking offers a chance to explore nature and challenge your body. Dancing can be a fun way to let loose and move to music. Both activities are enjoyable and great exercises. They don't feel like workouts because they're fun and social. You can share these experiences with friends or family, making them even more rewarding. Finding activities you love encourages you to keep moving and stay active in a way that feels natural.

Even the most minor actions can contribute to your fitness. Incidental exercise refers to the little bouts of activity scattered throughout your day. These are the moments when you choose the stairs over the elevator or take a brisk walk during your lunch break. Standing desks offer another way to incorporate movement into your routine. They encourage you to stand and stretch throughout the day, reducing the time spent sitting. These small efforts might not seem like much, but they add up. Studies show that even short bursts of movement can lower the risk of heart problems and improve overall health. Every move counts, and these small choices help build a healthier you.

Trying new activities keeps your routine fresh and exciting. It prevents boredom and challenges your body in new ways. Joining a local sports team or club connects you with others who share your interests. Playing sports not only keeps you fit but also builds friendships. You can learn new skills and enjoy the camaraderie of being part of a team. If you're looking for something different, try activities like rock climbing or kayaking. These offer adventure and test your strength and endurance. They push you out of your comfort zone and help you discover what your body can do. Exploring diverse activities keeps you engaged and makes fitness a fun part of life.

Sometimes, barriers can make staying active hard. Busy schedules and a lack of time can be significant obstacles. But there are ways to overcome them. Time management strategies help you find pockets of time for activity. Schedule short walks or do quick exercises during breaks. Even ten minutes of movement can boost your energy and improve your mood. Creating a home environment that encourages activity is another solution. Set up a space for exercise with equipment like weights or resistance bands. Keep your workout gear visible and accessible. This makes fitting activity into your day easier, even when life gets hectic.

By embracing movement as a lifestyle, you open the door to a healthier, more vibrant life. It's about making choices that fit your life and finding joy in moving. Instead of viewing exercise as a chore, see it as a way to enhance your well-being. The world becomes your gym, filled with opportunities to stay active and engaged. Whether it's a quick walk, a dance class, or a new sport, every movement brings you closer to a healthier you. Embrace the possibilities and let movement be a natural part of your day.

Step 1: Starting Position

🐦 Stand tall, setting an intention for the walk (e.g., "I will walk with awareness and control").

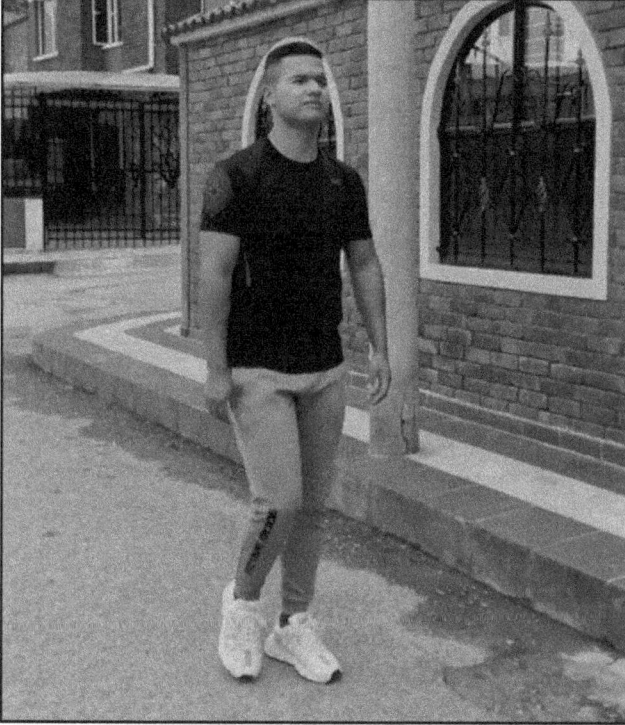

Step 2: Mindful Walking

🐦 Begin walking at a moderate pace, focusing on your breath and each step.

🐦 Inhale for 3 steps, then exhale for 3 steps. Maintain this pattern throughout the walk.

10.2 BUILDING A SUPPORTIVE COMMUNITY

Think about the last time you accomplished something difficult. It could be finishing a race or sticking to a new habit, and having someone cheer you on made a big difference. That's the power of community in fitness. You gain motivation and accountability when you connect with others who share your fitness goals. Local fitness groups or classes offer the chance to meet people who understand the challenges and triumphs of staying active. Whether it's a yoga class or a running club, being part of a group helps you stay committed. The encouragement and camaraderie you find in these settings can be the push you need to keep going.

In today's digital age, virtual communities offer similar benefits. Online forums and social media groups are excellent places to connect with like-minded individuals. You can share your experiences, ask questions, and get advice from people worldwide. These platforms break down barriers, allowing you to engage with others regardless of location. Many people find success by joining virtual fitness challenges. These challenges create a sense of belonging and friendly competition. They motivate you to push yourself further, knowing others are doing the same. Whether online or in person, being part of a fitness community provides the support and accountability that may be needed to stay on track.

Finding and building a fitness community doesn't have to be daunting. Start by attending local community events or workshops related to health and wellness. These events are great opportunities to meet people who share your interests. You might discover a new class or find a workout buddy. Engaging in online forums or social media groups also helps you connect with others. Look for groups that focus on your interests, whether hiking, weightlifting, or dance. Once you find your tribe, participate actively. Comment on posts, share your progress, and support others. Building relationships takes time, but your connections can become valuable to your fitness journey.

Shared fitness goals create strong bonds. Setting goals with others makes you more likely to stick to them. Organizing group challenges or competitions fosters a sense of camaraderie. It transforms fitness into a collective experience rather than a solitary task. For example, you might manage a friendly step-count competition with friends. Each person tracks their steps, and the group shares results weekly. This encourages physical activity and provides a fun way to engage with others. Sharing your progress and achievements with peers boosts motivation. Celebrating each other's successes builds a positive and supportive environment. Everyone wins when you cheer for others, and they cheer for you.

Maintaining supportive relationships requires effort but pays off. Regularly scheduling group workouts or meetups keeps the connection strong. Whether it's a Saturday morning run or a weekly fitness class, these gatherings provide a routine and structure. They hold you accountable and ensure you stay connected. Celebrating group milestones and successes is equally essential. When your group reaches a goal, celebrate together. This could be as simple as a group dinner or a shout-out on social media. Recognizing achievements reinforces the commitment to fitness and strengthens the bond among group members. It also reminds you of the progress made, reinforcing that you can achieve more together.

Creating and nurturing a supportive community transforms fitness from a chore into a shared adventure. The encouragement and accountability in these connections make it easier to stay committed. You find motivation not only in your progress but in the progress of others. This shared journey fosters a deep sense of belonging and purpose. Whether you meet in person or online, the relationships you build become a vital part of your fitness experience. They offer a network of support and motivation that keeps you moving forward, even when the path gets tough. Engaging with a fitness community opens you to new opportunities, experiences, and friendships that enhance your life in countless ways.

Step 1: Exercise 1 – Partner Squats

- Partner 1 performs a squat while Partner 2 provides support by holding Partner 1's arms.

- Partner 2 also performs the squat, using Partner 1's assistance for stability.

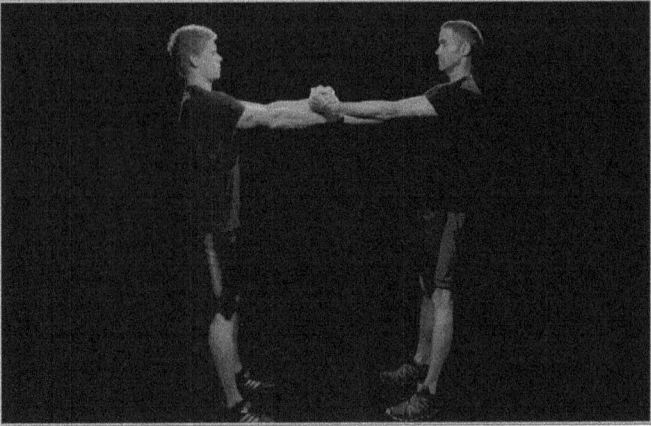

- Perform 10–12 reps together.

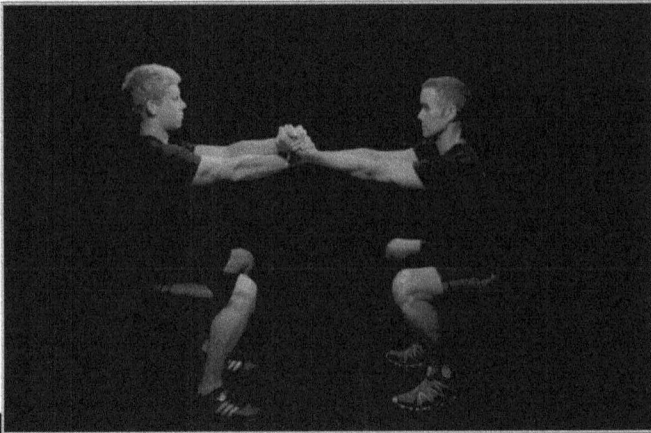

Step 2: Exercise 2 – Partner Leg Lifts

◦◦◦

➤ Partner 1 lies on their back with legs extended.

➤ Partner 2 assists by lifting Partner 1's legs while they engage their core to control the movement.

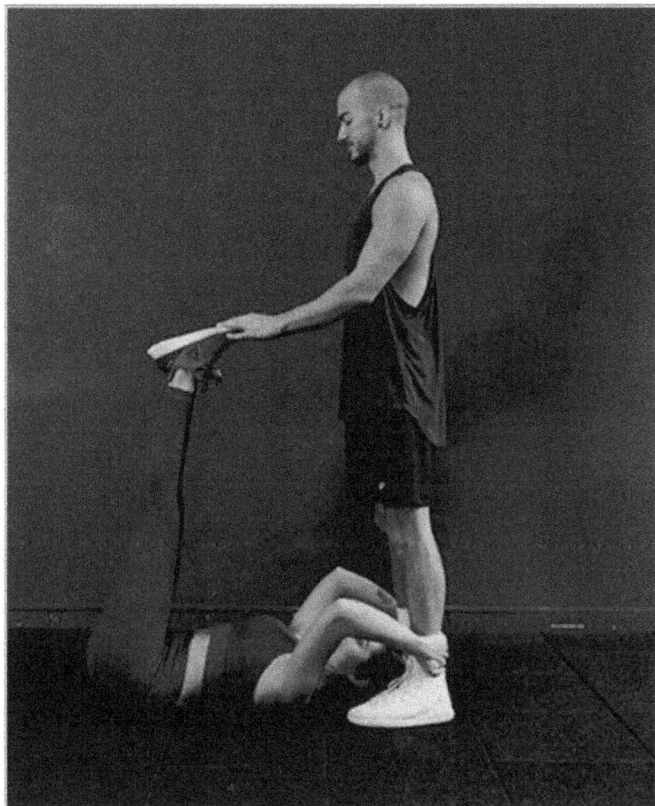

⟶ Perform 10-12 reps per leg.

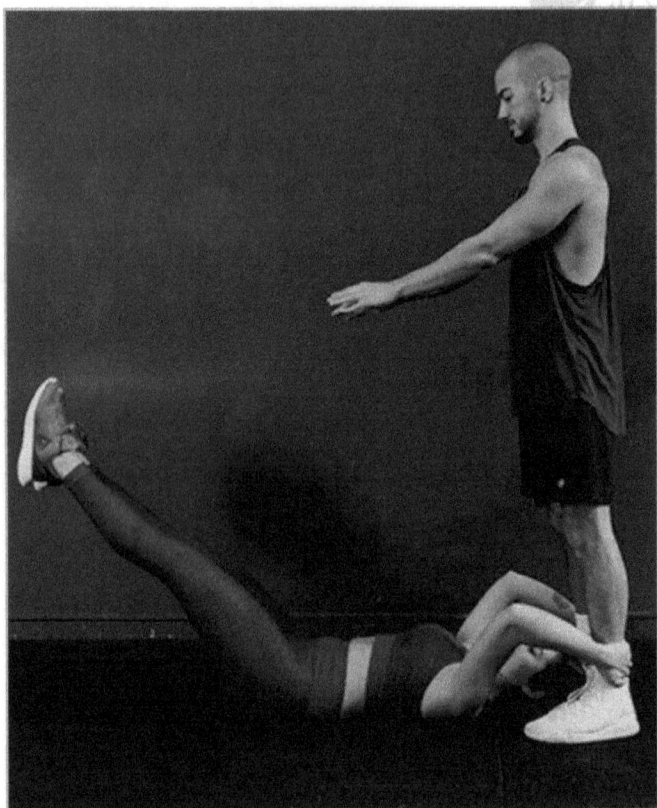

Step3: Cool Down

⟶ After completing the exercise, both partners perform a gentle stretch together to relax their muscles.

10.3 CONTINUING EDUCATION AND PROFESSIONAL GROWTH

In this ever-changing world of health and fitness, one truth stands firm: your journey never truly ends. Staying informed isn't just a helpful tool—it's your greatest ally. Knowledge is power, and by keeping up with the latest research, trends, and expert insights, you transform how you care for your mind and body.

Simple steps, like subscribing to reputable fitness magazines or journals, can keep you connected to the pulse of the industry. These resources bring fresh studies and expert perspectives right to your doorstep, sparking new ideas and keeping your motivation alive. With every article, you uncover strategies that elevate your daily routine, helping you make confident, informed decisions about your health.

Attending seminars and webinars opens even more doors. Imagine learning directly from top minds in nutrition, exercise science, and holistic wellness—asking questions, gaining new perspectives, and discovering breakthrough techniques you can start applying immediately. Whether it's a local seminar or a webinar replay you watch over coffee, these experiences make learning flexible, personal, and enriching.

For those in health or fitness professions, continuing education isn't just important—it's essential. Pursuing advanced certifications or training signals your dedication to excellence. It sharpens your expertise, expands your career opportunities, and connects you to a community of passionate peers and mentors who can guide and inspire you. The relationships you build through networking become pillars of support, collaboration, and fresh inspiration throughout your journey.

But formal education is only part of the equation. Self-exploration keeps your approach vibrant. Delving into new exercise methods or reading books by pioneers in holistic health challenges you to think bigger. These ideas stretch beyond the gym, exploring the profound connections between mind, body, and spirit. By trying new techniques and philosophies, you keep your routine from becoming stale, making each step on your journey exciting and meaningful.

And thanks to today's technology, expanding your knowledge has never been easier. Online platforms like Coursera and Udemy place a world of expertise at your fingertips, offering structured courses created by leading experts. Meanwhile, wellness workshops and retreats invite you to unplug, immerse yourself, and focus solely on growth, returning home refreshed, recharged, and brimming with new insights.

As you close this book, remember that learning is a lifelong adventure. Keep asking questions, stay curious, and never stop exploring. Each new skill you master, each concept you embrace, strengthens not only your body but your entire outlook on life.

So don't let your journey end here. Let this be the spark that propels you into a future of endless possibilities—because the best, most vibrant chapters of your life story are still waiting to be written.

Are you ready to turn the page?

THERAPEUTIC EXERCISES
SIMPLIFIED

You've made it! By now, you have the tools you need to move better, feel stronger, and take control of your health—one simple step at a time.

Whether you're just starting your journey or already feeling the benefits of therapeutic movement, this is just the beginning.

But now, **you can help someone else start their journey, too.**

By sharing your honest review on Amazon, you're not just giving feedback—you're showing other readers exactly where they can find the same clear, simple help that you did.

Your voice matters. And your review could be the *reason* someone picks up this book and starts believing in their body again.

With your help, we can reach:

- Parents are trying to stay active for their kids
- Older adults looking for gentle ways to stay mobile
- People recovering from injuries who want to feel strong again
- Anyone ready to feel better, but unsure where to begin

Thank you so much for being part of this journey. Therapeutic exercise is something we all deserve to understand—and when we pass on what we've learned, we keep that knowledge alive and growing.

👉 **Click here to leave your review on Amazon:**

https://www.amazon.com/review/create-review/?ie=UTF8&chan nel=glance-detail&asin=B0FM4MLFZL

With heartfelt thanks,

Solomon Cunningham

CONCLUSION

You've reached the end of our journey together. I'm so proud of you for taking this step towards a healthier, more vibrant life. Throughout this book, we've explored how therapeutic exercises are more than just a tool for recovery. It's a way to take control of your health and well-being. It's a path to lifelong strength, resilience, and vitality.

We've covered a lot of ground. We started by understanding the science behind therapeutic exercises, which helps your muscles grow stronger and your body move better. We then dove into the basics of building a strong foundation, focusing on factors such as core stability, range of motion, and proper alignment. These are the building blocks of safe and practical exercises.

Next, we talked about creating a personalized exercise plan. One that fits your unique needs and goals. You learned how to assess your starting point, set realistic targets, and track your progress. We also discussed the importance of listening to your body and making adjustments as needed.

We explored specific exercises tailored to various conditions, such as knee surgery recovery, hip replacement rehabilitation, and managing chronic pain. You discovered how to modify exercises to suit your needs. You also learned the value of patience and persistence in the healing process.

We delved into the world of motivation and mindset. You learned strategies for setting achievable goals, overcoming obstacles, and staying accountable. We also talked about the power of community and how having support can make all the difference.

But we didn't stop there. We looked at exercise from a holistic perspective. You discovered the importance of nutrition, sleep, and stress management in your overall health. We explored how practices like yoga and meditation can enhance your well-being. We also discussed ways to naturally incorporate movement into your daily life.

So, what now? It's time to take action. Start small. It could be a few stretches in the morning or a short walk after dinner. The key is to start and remain consistent. Remember, every little bit counts. As you incorporate exercise into your routine regularly, you'll begin to notice the benefits: more energy, a better mood, and a more substantial, more capable body.

Keep learning and growing. Stay curious about new ways to move and challenge yourself. Seek out information and inspiration from reliable sources. And don't be afraid to ask for help when you need it. Whether it's a friend, a family member, or a healthcare professional, having support can make the journey easier and more enjoyable.

Most importantly, believe in yourself. You have the power to transform your health and your life. It won't always be easy, but it will be worth it. Every step you take and every challenge you overcome is a testament to your strength and resilience.

Thank you for trusting me to guide you on this path. It's been an honor to share my knowledge and experience with you. This book has inspired you to see therapeutic exercises in a new light. Not just as a means to recover from injury or manage pain, but as a tool for unlocking your full potential.

Remember, movement is medicine. It's a gift that can heal, strengthen, and transform. Embrace it, and let it lead you to a life of vitality, joy, and endless possibilities.

Your partner in health,

[Solomon Cunningham]

REFERENCES

- *Therapeutic Exercise - StatPearls* https://www.ncbi.nlm.nih.gov/books/NBK555914/
- *De novo motor learning creates structure in neural activity ...* https://www.nature.com/articles/s41467-024-48008-7
- *Exercise therapy and mental health in clinical populations* https://www.cambridge.org/core/journals/advances-in-psychiatric-treatment/article/exercise-therapy-and-mental-health-in-clinical-populations-is-exercise-therapy-a-worthwhile-intervention/F73A667D4E5AE4484D8970EE7B86DF28
- *Exercising With Chronic Conditions | National Institute on Aging* https://www.nia.nih.gov/health/exercise-and-physical-activity/exercising-chronic-conditions
- *Why you should strengthen your core muscles* https://www.mayoclinic.org/healthy-lifestyle/fitness/in-depth/core-exercises/art-20044751
- *Range of Motion Exercises* https://www.benchmarkpt.com/blog/range-of-motion-exercises/
- *The effectiveness of proprioceptive training for improving ...* https://pmc.ncbi.nlm.nih.gov/articles/PMC4309156/
- *7 Foundational Functional Movements Key to Therapy & ...* https://moveperformance.com/2024/11/07/how-the-seven-foundational-functional-movements-are-the-key-to-physical-therapy-and-sports-performance-training/
- *Best Workout Apps for 2025* https://www.cnet.com/health/fitness/best-workout-apps/
- *Muscle Imbalance Explained (And 7 Ways to Improve It)* https://www.goodrx.com/conditions/musculoskeletal/fix-muscle-imbalance
- *How to set realistic fitness goals* https://www.precisionnutrition.com/how-to-set-realistic-fitness-goals
- *What to Use as Weights at Home | Home Workout Equipment* https://www.bicycling.com/skills-tips/g23451830/how-to-use-household-items-to-exercise-at-home/
- *Rehabilitation Techniques Before and After Total Knee ...* https://pmc.ncbi.nlm.nih.gov/articles/PMC10965116/
- *Hip Replacement Recovery: Guidelines, Tips, & Equipment* https://healthcare.utah.edu/orthopaedics/specialties/joint-replacement/patient-guide/after-hip-replacement#:~:text=Recovery%20for%20the%20First%20Three%20Months&text=Keep%20the%20surgical%20dressing%20over,cane%20when%20you%20feel%20ready.
- *Rotator Cuff and Shoulder Conditioning Program - OrthoInfo* https://orthoinfo.aaos.org/globalassets/pdfs/2017-rehab_shoulder.pdf
- *Physical activity and exercise for chronic pain in adults* https://pmc.ncbi.nlm.nih.gov/articles/PMC5461882/
- *Using Visuals in Physical Education: The Ultimate Guide ...* https://www.

capnpetespowerpe.com/single-post/using-visuals-in-physical-education-the-ultimate-guide-to-enhanced-learning-and-engagement-in-pe

- *5 Tips to Create Beautiful Fitness Infographics People Will ...* https://www.mypersonaltrainerwebsite.com/blog/5-tips-to-create-beautiful-fitness-infographics-people-will-love
- *How to Use QR Codes in Gyms and Fitness Products?* https://www.qrstuff.com/blog/general/how-to-use-qr-codes-in-gyms-and-fitness-products
- *The Best Workout Apps for 2025* https://www.pcmag.com/picks/best-workout-apps
- *How SMART Fitness Goals Can Help You Get Healthier* https://health.clevelandclinic.org/smart-fitness-goals
- *The Science & Psychology Of Goal-Setting 101* https://positivepsychology.com/goal-setting-psychology/
- *Fitness Accountability Partner - eVOLVSTRONG* https://evolvstrong.com/the-importance-of-a-fitness-accountability-partner-in-achieving-your-workout-goals/#:~:text=In%20an%20accountability%20partnership%2C%20effective,committed%20to%20your%20fitness%20routine.
- *Mindfulness exercises* https://www.mayoclinic.org/healthy-lifestyle/consumer-health/in-depth/mindfulness-exercises/art-20046356
- *Dynamic vs. Static Stretching: Is One Better?* https://health.clevelandclinic.org/dynamic-stretching-vs-static-stretching
- *Muscle Activation Exercises Prior To Training - [P]rehab* https://theprehabguys.com/muscle-activation/
- *5 Low Impact Cardio Exercises That Protect Your Joints* https://www.healthline.com/health/fitness-exercise/low-impact-exercises
- *7 Core Stability Exercises for Strength* https://www.acefitness.org/resources/everyone/blog/6313/7-core-stability-exercises/?srsltid=AfmBOorUuQpXhAdY9gNYegUrAMhgeCC7cj_ep_erOXteGrjKIcBln0g4
- *5 Tips for Exercising Safely While Rehabbing an Injury* https://www.houstonmethodist.org/blog/articles/2023/apr/5-tips-for-exercising-safely-while-rehabbing-an-injury/
- *Exercise Options for Limited Mobility* https://mhseniorliving.com/healthy-aging/stay-active-no-matter-what-exercise-options-for-those-with-limited-mobility/
- *Exercise and Activity in Pain Management* https://www.physio-pedia.com/Exercise_and_Activity_in_Pain_Management
- *Evaluating Online Exercise Information* https://eliteclubs.com/evaluating-online-exercise-information/
- *Nutrition and Muscle Recovery After Exercise - Frontiers* https://www.frontiersin.org/research-topics/54913/nutrition-and-muscle-recovery-after-exerciseundefined#:~:text=Nutrition%20plays%20a%20critical%20role,depends%20on%20energy%20substrate%20availability.
- *The importance of sleep for performance and recovery* https://www.hprc-online.org/physical-fitness/training-performance/importance-sleep-performance-and-recovery
- *Exercise for Mental Health - PMC* https://pmc.ncbi.nlm.nih.gov/articles/PMC1470658/

- *Yoga Therapy - Cleveland Clinic* https://my.clevelandclinic.org/health/treatments/24889-yoga-therapy#:~:text=Yoga%20therapy%20is%20a%20mind,treatment%20by%20a%20healthcare%20provider.
- *Habit Stacking: Helping Clients Achieve Results* https://www.trainerize.com/blog/habit-stacking/
- *Study pinpoints the length of incidental activity linked to ...* https://www.sydney.edu.au/news-opinion/news/2023/09/29/study-pinpoints-the-length-of-incidental-activity-linked-to-heal.html
- *How to build your online fitness community - AZEOO* https://azeoo.com/en/blog/how-to-build-your-online-fitness-community#:~:text=You%20can%20start%20by%20creating,help%20you%20build%20your%20community.
- *Therapeutic Exercise* https://www.physio-pedia.com/Therapeutic_Exercise

www.ingramcontent.com/pod-product-compliance
Lightning Source LLC
Chambersburg PA
CBHW031548260326
41914CB00002B/317